"Rachel Cosgrove is a writer who 'walks the walk.' An athlete, writer, and business owner, Rachel knows what it takes for women to be successful. I can guarantee you'll enjoy Rachel's book."

—*Mike Boyle, strength coach to numerous professional female athletes*

"Rachel Cosgrove is one of my top sources for fitness advice. She is, without a doubt, the best in the world at helping women lose fat and get in the best shape of their lives. In fact, there's no one in the fitness industry I trust more."

—*Adam Campbell, M.S., C.S.C.S., fitness director,* Men's Health

"I completed the 16-week [program] and my body is so different. I am smaller (and not just a smaller version of my old self!). I can't get over the reactions I get when people say, 'Boy, you must run a lot or do a lot of cardio.' It's truly amazing that I don't. I lift 'heavy,' *and* look better than ever. I love the fact that my arc trainer collects clothes in my basement and my stairs are getting the action. Thank you so much for writing a book that actually works!"

—*Megan Hoffman, fitness model,* Women's Health *cover model, bikini competitor*

"When it comes to getting real results for real women, I trust Rachel Cosgrove. She is hands down one of the best female trainers in the country, and I wouldn't want anyone else as our fitness columnist at *Women's Health.* She understands that women today want to look great, but have less time and motivation than ever. Her approach is realistic and motivating, and her book is filled with all the tools to positively push women to results they never thought possible. If you want to change your body (and your life!) for good, read this book."

—*Jen Ator, fitness editor,* Women's Health *magazine*

"If you really need elite training and superior results, you need to go to Results Fitness. It is not only top in cutting-edge functional equipment, but the staff is for real. The owners—Rachel and Alwyn—are among the few in the industry who demand that their trainers go through real education and training before they even begin to teach or work with anyone. Not only are they knowledgeable, but they are also friendly and dedicated to producing results with their clientele. In addition, I can say with confidence that one of the owners, Rachel, is at par with me when it comes to nutrition. So if you want it all—performance, nutrition, knowledge, and support—you must visit Results Fitness."

—*Dr. Eric Serrano, M.D. Dr. Serrano earned his medical degree from the University of Kansas and is Board Certified in Family Medicine. In addition to his clinical practice, Dr. Serrano also serves as a nutritional and medical consultant to elite and professional athletes around the world.*

"I have had the pleasure of knowing Rachel Cosgrove both as a friend and a colleague for many years now. Most people who know me know that I, #1 don't give too many testimonials, and #2 rarely call someone the 'real deal.' Rachel Cosgrove is the real deal, period. As a conditioning coach training people to meet their fitness goals, as an athlete competing in powerlifting and triathlons, to being one of the most well-respected professionals in this industry who constantly provides continuing education for others in this field, Rachel is pretty much the total package. In an industry dominated by males and more testosterone than one would like, Rachel stands out as a female who will hold her own with any of us in this field."

— *Robert dos Remedios, M.A., C.S.C.S., S.C.C.C. 2006 NSCA Collegiate Strength and Conditioning Professional of the Year; Director of Speed, Strength and Conditioning, College of the Canyons, California Author of* Men's Health Power Training

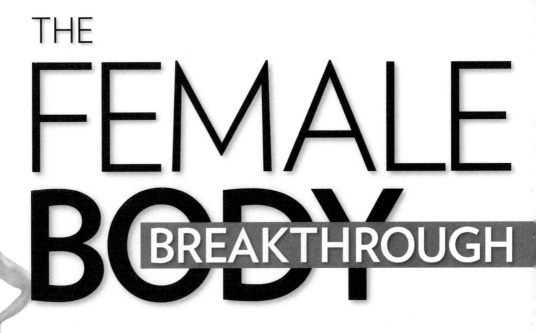

THE
FEMALE
BODY
BREAKTHROUGH

THE REVOLUTIONARY STRENGTH-TRAINING PLAN FOR LOSING FAT AND **GETTING THE BODY YOU WANT**

RACHEL COSGROVE, BS, CSCS

RODALE

This book is dedicated to my niece, Marie Osborn.
Her strong spirit, determination, and nothing-will-hold-her-back
attitude inspire me every day in everything I do.

© 2009 by Rachel Cosgrove
Photographs (Illustrations) © 2009 by Rodale Inc.

Rodale books may be purchased for business or promotional use or for special sales. For information, please write to:
Special Markets Department, Rodale, Inc., 733 Third Avenue, New York, NY 10017

Printed in the United States of America
Rodale Inc. makes every effort to use acid-free ⊗, recycled paper ♻.

Photographs © Mitch Mandel/Rodale Images
Book design by Christina Gaugler

Library of Congress Cataloging-in-Publication Data
Cosgrove, Rachel.
    The female body breakthrough : the revolutionary strength-training plan for losing fat and getting the body you want / Rachel Cosgrove.
        p.   cm.
    Includes bibliographical references and index.
    ISBN-13 978–1–60529–693–7 pbk.
    ISBN-10 1–60529–693–7 pbk.
    1. Weight loss—Psychological aspects.   2. Women—Health and hygiene.   3. Physical fitness for women.   I. Title.
RM222.2.C646   2009
613.2'5—dc22   2009036098

Distributed to the trade by Macmillan
2   4   6   8   10   9   7   5   3   1   paperback

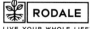

We inspire and enable people to improve their lives and the world around them
For more of our products visit **rodalestore.com** or call 800-848-4735

Contents

Introduction

✦ You've tried every diet and weight-loss program and have failed to achieve the body you want.

✦ You've lost weight in the past, only to gain it right back. You have had (or have come painfully close to having) the body you wanted, but it was only temporary.

✦ You have a closet full of clothes you can't fit into. But you keep them in hopes that one day you will fit into them again. You call them your "skinny clothes."

✦ You try on at least three different outfits every time you get ready to go somewhere, because you don't like the way you look in any of them. This one shows every bulge and dimple, that one accentuates your muffin top, and you feel like your butt looks huge in all of them. Then you finally settle on something baggy and probably black because it's supposed to be slimming and you think it hides everything, but it really just makes you look bigger.

✦ You hate seeing pictures of yourself and hide when someone takes out a camera. You are consistently the floating head in the back of a group photo.

✦ You want the lights off when you and your significant other are getting busy.

✦ You are always tired and never have energy.

✦ Your sex drive is in the gutter.

✦ You look with envy at confident women with great bodies who are comfortable in their own skin, but you think you could never look like that.

✦ You're self-conscious about your body and don't like to draw attention to yourself.

✦ You don't work out at a gym because you're intimidated; or if you do, you stick to the cardio machines in the corner because, again, you don't want to draw attention to yourself.

✦ Maybe you think of yourself as the "fat" friend among your peers. That's who you are, and that's who you think you'll always be.

If none of these sound like you, then maybe you're already fit and confident. Congratulations! But even you could learn a thing or two from this book, or at least get an extra dose of motivation!

Listen up, ladies! I'm your coach, and my goal is to help you to make the breakthrough to become a fit and fabulous female. I'm going to talk to you girl to girl, woman to woman, or I guess we should say fit female to fit female! Since it's just us girls talking, I want to talk to you a little bit about this journey we are about to embark on together and let you know that throughout this book I will be pushing you outside your comfort zone. I will challenge you to think differently about exercise, nutrition, and your body. I will be very candid, open, and honest, and I'll even share my own story of my journey to fitness. In return, I need you to be honest and up front with me and with yourself. This book and this challenge is a safe place for you to let go of any negative thoughts you have about your body or your ability to create the body you want. I want you to embrace a whole new you. Don't hold back, and neither will I. If you're reading this book right now, you are committing to making a change and following through with the advice within these pages to make the breakthrough to become a fit, confident female.

I've filled these pages with honest, candid stories of my own journey to finding my own fit female body and those of the spectacular women I've trained in the gym I co-own with my husband in Southern California. I want these stories to inspire you to write your own story of transformation. All I ask for in return is your commitment to write a new story for yourself by following the plan in this book. Remember to enjoy the metamorphosis—the journey is just as important as the end result.

So who is this fit female, anyway? You know the girl . . . the one at the last party you went to who walked in the room feeling sexy and confident in her flirty black dress without a roll or a bulge in sight and worked the room with her confidence, looking fabulous! At the time, you may have referred to her as "that bitch who walked in the room thinking she is somebody," and you might have wondered who she thought she was. But deep down we all know she has what all of us want: She feels sexy and confident in her own skin and has the killer body we have all dreamed of having. A true fit female has confidence in herself. When someone compliments her on her body, she does not reply, "Oh my god! You must be joking! I'm huge!" Instead, she knows how to take a compliment, because she feels good about herself. She is the girl every woman wants to be and every man wants to be with. She is fit and fabulous. From now on, *BITCH* stands for **B**e Inspiring, **T**otally **C**onfident, and **H**ot! Don't envy her—become the **BITCH**! If you resent what someone has, you will never have it. Instead, be inspired and become that person.

You may also have seen her in the grocery store or at a restaurant. She was wearing a tank top and jeans, looking fit and confident, or maybe she was in her workout clothes. You've seen her a couple of times, and every single time she looks in shape, never bloated or having a fat day. Her arms have definition, her tummy is flat, and you could bounce a quarter off her butt. Nothing jiggles or wiggles. You can tell she works out—there is no question. You may even be asking yourself what sport she plays or what kind of athlete she is. Most important, she is totally confident in her body and feels good about herself. She looks so good that when you first saw her, you probably did a double take because you don't see women like this very often. A fit female is empowered, fit, and sexy. Her confidence in herself is what makes her sexy. She has the type of body that makes you say, "*That* is what I want to look like." Once this book is released and more women get their hands on it and start to follow the advice within, this fit female will become a more common sight. Why can't you be the one people are pointing at, saying, "*That* is what I want to look like." You can!

"It's not who you are that holds you back; it's who you think you're not."

—UNKNOWN

This book is your guide to becoming fit, confident, and empowered. Think of it as your fit body manual. You should not read this book once, put it on your shelf, and be done with it. Instead, make it your constant companion.

Read through it a few times, make notes in it, circle or highlight quotes or stories that inspire you. Write down thoughts that you have as you read it, and add sticky notes earmarking the chapters you know you'll want to refer back to. When you hit an obstacle or have a week when you're struggling to stay on track with your program, go back to certain chapters and reread the information. Use it as your very own coach to keep you focused and motivated.

Within these pages I will do everything I can to turn each and every one of you into a fit female, feeling empowered, sexy, confident, and fabulous! Actually, starting today, from this moment on, think of yourself as a fit female in training—on your way to a killer bod!

Within these pages you will reinvent yourself. First you will find the Fit Female Credo, which will give you the rules to live by as a fit female in training. Get these basic rules down and live by them every single day. Reread this credo on a regular basis. Then you will learn how to start your reinvention; don't skip this section of the book! You'll also find exactly what you need to do in the gym to become fit and empowered. The training program and nutrition program have four different phases lasting four weeks each, to transition you into being a fit female.

+ Phase One: **Base phase** to clean up your diet, correct imbalances, and give you a base strength. This is the phase you'll come back to throughout the year to maintain your fit female body. This is home base.

✦ Phase Two: **Define yourself phase** to build some definition, get your metabolism revving, and learn how to splurge without feeling guilty.

✦ Phase Three: **Dial it in phase** to really burn some calories, continue building strength, learn to time your carbohydrates, and completely change the way you look.

✦ Phase Four: **Fine-tune phase,** in which you'll really push yourself to peak and become the BITCH. This phase is tough but is meant to help you peak for an event or goal. **Be** Inspiring, **T**otally **C**onfident and **H**ot!

The programs in this book are not limited to 16 weeks but instead can be revisited depending on where you are in your journey, with tweaks in the intensity and load to get your metabolism revving. That is the goal of the workouts in this book: to boost your metabolism and turn you into a fat-burning machine. The plans in this book have all been tested. They have been used in my gym with actual clients, some of whom are featured in the book. I've fine-tuned the strategies by working with more than a thousand women, including myself, to create fit females. Even the model in this book has done the program. You will never be lost in the gym without a plan again. Along with all this, I will share my journey and many of my clients' journeys with you, for you to connect with, be inspired by, and learn from. You'll also get every tidbit of information, every tool, and every

quote I have used with my clients in the gym. You'll know every secret! You'll even speak the fit female language and find yourself saying things like "eating clean," "state of total starvation," "training hard," and "dialing it in." You'll hear this language in the real life stories throughout this book.

This book is about becoming empowered and never feeling self-conscious about your body again. This book gives women permission to feel confident and good about their bodies. You'll notice that the before and after pictures of my clients show women of all shapes and sizes changing their bodies and feeling empowered, fit, and sexy—they each have a different fit female body! It's not about fitting a mold; it's about finding your best fit female body and feeling absolutely fabulous! It's about changing the way women work out, eat, and feel about their bodies. You will challenge yourself in the gym, gaining strength and lean muscle, boosting your metabolism, fueling your body, and becoming the confident, fit woman you've always wanted to become for life. You will inspire others!

You have everything you need in this manual to become fit, confident, and empowered. As you are transforming yourself with this book, another resource for you is the website I set up to connect you with other fit females, thefemalebodybreakthrough.com. Stay connected and motivated, and make this a change for the long term.

Make your "someday" TODAY!

Part 1

WHAT'S THE FIT FEMALE CHALLENGE ABOUT?

Chapter 1

The Fit Female Credo

Breakthrough Secrets to Becoming Fit and Fabulous for Life

What secrets does a fit female know that you don't? How do you become the BITCH? Become Inspiring, Totally Confident, and Hot. The following is the Fit Female Credo, which includes the "goods" when it comes to knowing what to do and how to behave to turn yourself into a fit female for life. These are the real cues, visualizations, and tools I share with my clients on a daily basis to help them stay focused on their goal. I am going to let you in on every strategy, trick, and secret that you need to know to become fit and fabulous. There are 168 hours in a week, and I am with my clients on average only two to three of those hours; the rest of the week they are on their own (like you, the readers of this book). I have to arm them with the ammo to survive whatever life might throw at them and whatever difficult situation they may encounter. No matter what progress we make during the two to three hours I'm with them, if I don't equip them with tools for the rest of the week, they can do a lot of damage in the 166 hours they're on their own. This credo contains your rules to live by every single day to turn yourself into a fit, confident woman.

In this chapter, I'll discuss how to live the lifestyle of a fit female, get your head in the right place, surround yourself with supportive people, make time for fitness, and once and for all stop making excuses! Everyone has an excuse. There will always be one. I don't want to hear it! Stop blaming someone else or something else for not being where you want to be. Instead, take on the challenge and take ownership of every choice you make. One of these secrets may be the breakthrough you need to finally change your mind, your body, and your life. Listen up!

FIT FEMALE CREDO
Secret #1: Act as if you are a fit female.

Don't wait until 10 pounds from now—start being one today. You must start to live like a fit female now in order to become one. You must act like one, eat like one, talk like one, dress like one. When you see what happens when you start acting as if you are a fit female, you will become one before you know it. This may sound silly, but I've seen it work for so many of my clients. The mind-body connection is more powerful than you think. I have seen women lose weight and change their bod-

ies, only to gain the weight back again. On the other hand, I've seen other women lose weight, change their bodies, and become fit and empowered for life. What was the difference? The difference was that the ones who succeeded changed their mindsets and saw themselves as fit females. They acted fit and confident, they dressed in tighter clothes to show off their new bodies, and they felt empowered. The ones who did not succeed and gained the weight back never really thought of themselves as being fit and fabulous and having the body they always wanted. They couldn't picture it, and even when they had it, they couldn't see it, but still saw themselves as fat and frumpy. They still wore baggy clothes, covered themselves up, and did not feel confident, even though their bodies had completely transformed. They ended up gaining the weight back because they had always seen themselves as having the extra weight. It is just as important to transform your mind as it is to transform your body. Use the visualization tool I talk about in Chapter 4, Deciding What You Want and Why. It works. Be a fit female starting today. Remember, make your "someday" today!

In the real life story that follows, my client, Haley, wore a baggy T-shirt and long sweats to work out on day one. I made her roll up her shirt so we could see what she looked like, but she was in her frumpy mindset, wearing baggy clothes, trying to hide what was underneath. By the end, for her after picture, she walked

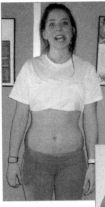

▲
Haley before

Haley as a fit female ▶

Haley lost 20 pounds of fat and 4 jean sizes.

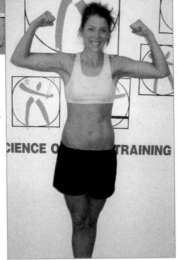

FIT FEMALE *Real Life Story*

Even as a high school athlete, I never lifted weights. I thought practice was enough to get me in shape and that the occasional suicide I ran for punishment would give me those desired runner's legs. But that definitely wasn't the case, and I don't need to tell you that, because my body reflected it.

I was new to lifting and had never done any sort of weight training. But it quickly became a part of my lifestyle, and I have never been able to shake it. My athleticism skyrocketed, and because of it, I received a full-ride volleyball scholarship. Along with my coaches and even my athletic director, I credited my changes as an athlete to the strength programs I was doing. I have been a standout player since I was a freshman, and because of the hard work I put in, I've been able accomplish some pretty far-fetched goals.

But in the process of working toward athletic success, I achieved something that I never thought I would find: confidence. Like most young adults, I had always been very insecure in my own skin. But I eventually started seeing small changes in my body every time I looked in the mirror. But that was only when I was lifting and I hadn't yet incorporated any nutrition. When I started meeting with Rachel about nutrition, I realized how naive I'd been to think that the two (working out and eating right) didn't go hand in hand. We put together some menus that correlated with my workouts, and before my eyes, the fat started melting away. It was a long and hard process; but, with the right tools, it became much easier. The same way that lifting weights had become a lifestyle, so had eating right.

I lost 20 pounds and gained about eight pounds of pure muscle. I was a better athlete, but more important, I was confident. I left to go to college as a young woman who felt confident and sexy. And here I am five years later with the same confidence. But the most empowering thing of all was that I gave this gift of feeling confident to myself, using weight training and nutrition to fuel my body. ✦

into the gym wearing this—a sports bra and short shorts. Besides just seeing the 20 pounds of fat gone, Haley had a whole new self-confidence, and it showed in the way she dressed and the way she felt about her body.

"If we don't change, we don't grow. If we don't grow, we aren't really living."

—GAIL SHEEHY

Secret #2: Get out of your comfort zone!

To get your body to change, you have to do what your body is not used to. This may mean taking yourself outside of your comfort zone. Your comfort zone is where things are easy—they don't feel like work or like an effort. Guess what—if it seems easy and comfortable, you probably aren't going to transform your body. To prompt your body to change, you have to make it do what it's not used to. This means the foods you eat will take some effort to plan and prepare (and if your schedule is busy, that may not come easily), the training you do will feel challenging, and you'll be pushing yourself beyond what you're used to. If you don't feel like you have to go against your usual routine, then you probably are not going to change your body. You have to do something different from what you're currently doing to push your body to change. Get used to going outside of your comfort zone and challenging yourself to do it on a daily basis. I

didn't say this would be really hard or unbearable, just outside of your usual comfort zone. Learn to enjoy that feeling of challenging yourself to shake things up.

So change your routine. If your usual routine is to come home from work and lounge on the couch with your favorite food, mindlessly noshing, checking out from your day by watching TV, get out and do something or go to the gym instead. Go for a walk, call up a supportive friend, or write in your journal. Your habits can easily be changed, starting now. Think about what habits you have that are keeping you from becoming that confident fit girl you want to be. Act like a fit female and you will become a fit female. Change your habits as of today!

People will do almost anything to stay in their comfort zones. If you want to accomplish anything, get out of your comfort zone. Strive to increase order and discipline in your life. Discipline usually means doing the opposite of what you feel like doing.

—DAVE KEKICH

Secret #3: Fuel your body to be fabulous!

Eat more often, not less. Becoming fit and fabulous is not about starving yourself and feeling deprived. The key is to get your metabolism revving, fuel your body throughout the day with healthy foods, and learn how to enjoy a guilt-free splurge that fits into your healthy

CATABOLIC:

A scientific term for the state your body goes into when you don't fuel it every couple of hours and it starts to break down hard-earned muscle tissue. Being catabolic is detrimental to your physique. You want to avoid being catabolic at all costs. Used in a sentence: "I need to eat before I become catabolic!" Never let your body become catabolic.

lifestyle. To obtain a fit, fabulous body free of cellulite and belly fat, you must fuel your body with unprocessed whole foods every couple of hours to rev your metabolism. Instead of starving your body and letting your metabolism stall out, creating an ideal situation to gain the weight back, the goal is to fuel your body and boost your metabolism to the point where your body burns through the food you eat and you have to continue fueling it to keep your metabolism revving. You work very hard in the gym to change your body; you have to fuel it to keep it, or you'll become catabolic.

Secret #4: Train hard or go home!

A fit female is not afraid of lifting challenging weights and pushing herself in the gym. She sweats, she grunts, and she puts demands on her body that are outside of her comfort zone, keeping her muscles challenged, defined, and strong and giving her a sizzling metabolism. She looks the way she does *because she has muscle,* the very thing you may be afraid of building. The secret to getting your metabolism

revving high enough to melt away fat to become a fit female is the type of workouts you do. A recent study compared weight lifting to aerobics. Both groups lost 26 pounds on the scale, but the group who did strength training lost only fat, while the aerobics group lost 8 percent of their weight from muscle. Losing muscle slows down your metabolism. The priority workout for a fit female is one that boosts her metabolism, burns calories, builds muscle, and creates an afterburn effect. The best workout to accomplish this is strength training, and the key is to challenge yourself in the gym, pushing your intensity. Less is more when it comes to exercise. Don't be afraid to lift heavier weights to eke out your last rep, challenging yourself to train hard. Fit, confident females don't bother with 3-pound dumbbells, aerobics, endless cardio, or machines in the gym.

Secret #5: Get hooked on feeling fit, not the number on the scale!

Be your own inspiration. Being fit is motivating, and the feeling is addicting. If you can tap into the sensation of being confident, fit, empowered, and sexy and really tune in to how that feels, you'll do anything to get that. Forget the scale and experience this feeling instead.

I constantly see this transformation in the gym, from women wearing baggy T-shirts, standing with slumped shoulders, and feeling really self-conscious to wearing tight-fitting clothes, buying new outfits all the time, and feeling confident and sexy. One of my clients, after losing 40 pounds of fat, said, "I love to go shopping for clothes again. I never used to wear tank tops, and now that's all I wear." When I talked to one of my clients about her transformation, she described it as a "high." And she said the feeling is addicting! This is when it clicked for me that you have to get hooked on this feeling to be successful. She talked about how she used to go home from work and put on her baggiest sweats and T-shirt to do things around the house. Now she struts her stuff in her boy shorts and tank top feeling so confident about herself and addicted to that feeling. Her husband isn't complaining, either.

If you have ever had your ideal body in the past, think back to how great you felt. Visualize this feeling right when you start your challenge. Picture yourself there and recall how you felt. As your body changes—and as you're shopping for new clothes—you will feel so amazing you'll never want that feeling to go away. No sugary food or salty treat tastes as good as lean and sexy feels. It is like a high, and it is addicting. Find the motivation within and feed off it every single day. A fit female does not focus on the scale but instead focuses on how she looks in her clothes and how she feels. This is what inspires and motivates her to keep going and stay on track!

Secret #6: Be an early riser.

Get up early and start your day with a workout. This will set up your day for success. I am a big believer in morning workouts. Doing some form of exercise first thing in the morning will psychologically set you up to succeed for the day while getting your metabolism cranking so you can continue to burn fat throughout the day. This will also eliminate the chance of anything else getting in the way of your workout, and you'll give it 100 percent energy instead of just giving it whatever energy is left over at the end of the day. Remember, you'll never regret working out, but you'll always regret it if you don't. Doing your workout first thing in the morning will ensure that you don't have any regrets! Be sure to eat some breakfast beforehand and finish with a postworkout shake.

"Early to bed, early to rise makes a man healthy, wealthy, and wise!"

—BENJAMIN FRANKLIN

Secret #7: Make R, R, & R a priority!

You don't just need R & R. . . . You need R, R, & R—rest, relaxation, and regeneration. When you're pushing your body daily with intense workouts, reward yourself and regenerate by getting your rest and relaxation. You're asking a lot of your body; give back to it. Finish your day with something relaxing, such as stretching, reading a good book, writing in a journal, or enjoying a bubble bath with candles and relaxing music. Take time each day to do something for yourself. You deserve it! Rewarding yourself will also keep you motivated. This is a great time to visualize and get refocused on exactly what you want to accomplish, who you want to become, and what your goals are. Take time each day to do this.

Also be sure to get at least 6 to 8 hours of shut-eye a night. Getting enough sleep is extremely important to your recovery and your results. Do not skimp on your sleep. Research has shown that as sleep quality and quantity decrease, levels of the stress hormone cortisol (which we'll talk more about in Secret #13) increase, while levels of growth hormone, a hormone linked to building muscle and burning fat, decrease. This is not the optimal situation to build a fit female body. Plus, less time awake means less time to gobble down ice cream, chips, or whatever else you usually have as a midnight snack. No more midnight rendezvous with the fridge. Go to bed. Being sleep deprived will lead to low energy, ineffective workouts, cravings for sugar for quick energy, and a cycle of behavior that will take you further away from your fit body.

A fit female understands the concept that she does not build her fit female body during the workout—she builds it when she recovers from the workout. Taking time off to regenerate is one of the keys to building a fit female body. More is not better if you're not recovering. Get your sleep, take some downtime, and reward yourself with some R, R & R every day.

Secret #8: Obstacles will arise—anticipate them!

"You may have a fresh start any moment you choose, for this thing we call 'failure' is not the falling down, but the staying down."

—Mary Pickford

You will undoubtedly have obstacles throughout your journey. When they show up, don't let them throw you too far off track. Successful people see obstacles as opportunities to be challenged and to learn about themselves. You should feel the same way. Tell yourself you will stay focused and keep yourself on track. You may get sick or injured, or maybe a family member will get sick or you'll have a family emergency. Everyone has obstacles—everyone! Working with clients, I hear stories of all kinds of obstacles, and sometimes it may mean a setback, but don't let it completely derail you from reaching your goal. Stay focused on what you want and why you want it, and that focus will pull you through your obstacles like a magnet. Knowing that they will show up and that you will have to deal with them will make the surprise of their arrival easier to deal with, so take them on as a challenge! And when you're on the other side of each one, you'll be so glad you got through it while keeping yourself focused on what you ultimately want for yourself. Remember, the journey is as important as reaching the destination.

Fit Female Visual Tool

I have heard that when a pilot is flying a plane, the course is never a direct straight line from point A to point B. Instead, the pilot must always make small adjustments to the direction the plane is going in order to stay on the right path to the destination. This is exactly how your journey will be. It won't be a straight line, but instead you may have obstacles come up that send you off the path, or you may think you are on track but then realize you need to make a change to get where you're going. Focus on making small changes one at a time, and if an obstacle bumps you off track, make an adjustment and steer yourself back again, but keep moving forward, visualizing your destination and what it will feel like. Eventually you will land at your destination and will be fit and fabulous.

One obstacle that often arises is coming down with a bug. You are motivated and consistent with your training and nutrition, and then wham, you get hit with a flu bug or other illness. You may be so focused and motivated that you feel as if you should keep training right through the sickness, but this will only set you back further. Here's the deal: When you work out, your body makes repairing your muscles and recovering the No. 1 priority. But when you're sick, the priority becomes fighting off whichever bug you've caught. Recovering from your workout gets put on the back burner; exercising gives your body one more thing to put energy toward and will usually prolong the sickness by keeping your body from fighting off the bug. The rule is this: When you're sick, take a break and let your body rest so it can fight off whatever you have. This way you'll be able to come back sooner and feel good enough to hit your workouts hard again. Also, when you do a workout, your immune system weakens temporarily and then afterward rebuilds itself stronger. Again, this is not an ideal situation when your body is already fighting off an illness. Take a break and let your body fight. You'll be back in no time and better than ever!

Secret #9: Keep a journal or blog.

"A life worth living is worth recording!"

—JIM ROHN

Choose a journal you like to write in and fill it with motivational sayings, pictures, or anything that keeps you focused. If you prefer the Doogie Howser/Carrie Bradshaw method, get in front of a computer and start a blog. Keeping up a blog will hold you accountable when people start to read and comment on it. Write down your goals and put them in your journal, where you'll see them every day. You should at least be keeping track of your meals and work-outs and how you feel—energized, tired, motivated, etc. This will make you conscious of your habits, your mood, your energy, what's working, and most importantly, what isn't working.

Secret #10: Eliminate the crabs and surround yourself with supportive people.

I went crabbing once in Seattle, and we went out in a boat and dropped big crab traps down in the water with markers on them. We left them there all day and later that day went back out and pulled them up full of crabs.

We took them to shore and put all the crabs in a big open bucket of water. Surprisingly, all the crabs stayed in the bucket and did not climb out, even though it was wide open. We left the crabs in this open bucket all night long. If one crab tried to climb out of the bucket, the other crabs would pull him back down, and if he continued to try to climb out, the other crabs would pull one of his legs off and make sure to keep him in the bucket. This was so interesting, since you'd think the other crabs would instead realize that if one of them could climb out, they too could escape. But instead they were more interested in keeping everyone in the bucket. It is amazing how closely this reflects human nature. When someone is doing something to become more successful or to better themselves, whether it's to start an exercise program or eat more healthily, other people will try to drag that person back down to their level and keep them from being successful. After all, if that person succeeds, it will make everyone else look bad. Instead of joining in and making the same positive changes, human nature seems to be to bring that person back down.

This analogy can be extremely helpful when you're trying to make a change in your life. For example, when you're out to dinner with friends and everyone is giving you a hard time about not ordering alcohol or not eating the basket of bread, and they're telling you, "Just have one drink!" Or maybe when you want to have an early night because you have to be up early the next morning to get your workout done and everyone pressures you, saying, "You can miss one workout!" If you've ever tried to make a drastic change, you have experienced this aspect of human nature and will continue to experience it, but next time, you can simply think in your head that your friends are all just a bunch of crabs!

Don't let their negative words get to you. They can be poisonous to your success.

"I believe that you should gravitate to people who are doing positive and productive things with their lives."

—NADIA COMANECI

You have to surround yourself with people who will support you in your quest to transform yourself. I've seen it so many times: A client comes in with a drive to change her body and feel good, but her husband or someone in her immediate circle is constantly sabotaging her with negative comments and keeping her from succeeding—he's being a crab. On the other hand, a supportive husband or significant other can be extremely powerful in helping a woman achieve success with her fitness goals. All he needs to say is, "Wow! Babe, you are looking amazing!" and she has all the motivation she needs to keep pushing herself to look and feel even better.

Ask yourself these questions: "Who is in my immediate circle? Are they supportive, or are they crabs? Are they sucking the motivation out of me?"

Where do you fit in? Are you a crab? If you find that you are, don't be discouraged. Instead, decide you will change. Not only will you become fit and fabulous, but you'll also become an uplifting, supportive person to be around, with a passion for living life to the absolute fullest and inspiring others. You will be the BITCH (in a positive sense, of course).

Start to be conscious of whom you spend your time with. Eliminate any negative, "poor me"-thinking people (also known as crabs) from your life and surround yourself with supportive, positive people. If those around you are feeding you negative thoughts, it will be nearly impossible to undo that and have success. Negative thoughts are poison to your success as a fit, confident female.

"To attract attractive people, you must be attractive. To attract powerful people, you must be powerful. To attract committed people, you must be committed. Instead of going to work on them, you go to work on yourself. If you become, you can attract."

—Jim Rohn

Secret #11: Think about your thoughts.

This goes along with the last secret and your becoming an uplifting, positive person, eliminating any negative, poisonous thoughts and people from your life. Throughout your day, pay attention to the dialogue you use in your head, everything you are thinking or saying to yourself. If a negative and self-deprecating thought or picture enters your mind, immediately substitute one that is motivating and supportive to what you want to accomplish. Would a fit female think that about herself? As long as you're talking negatively to yourself, you will not become an empowered, confident fit female. Every thought you have will either empower you or disempower you. You must change your mindset and your internal dialogue so that the only messages you send yourself are those that can empower you. The one thing you have absolute control over is your mindset. Changing your lifestyle and improving your fitness are about making small changes that will eventually lead to reaching your goal, and it starts with immediately changing your thoughts. This takes practice.

Start to be more conscious and "think about your thoughts" and how they may be affecting who you are and who you're becoming. You have only so many thoughts each day, and you can't afford to waste any on negative ones. It isn't worth it. According to the National Science Foundation, you are bombarded with about 50,000 thoughts a day.

"You are exactly what you believe and think about all day long. Constantly monitor your thoughts."

—UNKNOWN

Secret #12: Attitude is everything!

"If you don't like something, change it. If you can't change it, change your attitude."

—MAYA ANGELOU

Just like in the song you used to belt out with the Pointer Sisters—"I got a new attitude!"—attitude is a choice, and you can choose to have a new attitude at any time. Make that choice! Your attitude toward fitness will determine whether this will be a lifestyle change. If

Fit Female Visual Tool

You are your own computer programmer! You have the ability to write the computer program that will create the person you want to become. You have about 50,000 commands (thoughts) to send to your computer (brain) every day. If you use the right commands, they will program you to become fit, confident, and empowered female. Every thought you have is another programming message to your brain instructing it, just like a computer, to tell your body to behave a certain way. The one thing you have *total* control over is every thought you let enter your head, and therefore what you program your brain to tell your body to become. You must program your brain that you are fit and fabulous in order to become fit female. Be aware of how you talk to yourself and what you think to yourself daily. Every thought is a message taking you closer to becoming the person you want to become or farther away. You are programming yourself, and you have total control. Whenever you become aware of a repetitive negative thought or programming message, ask yourself: Are you giving your body the commands it needs to create the program to become the person you want to become? Are you using your 50,000 commands a day to create a fit, confident, empowered woman?

your attitude toward fitness is that it's too hard, time consuming, and not worth it, you'll never make it a priority, and it will never become a lifestyle. It is true that the mind and body are connected, and if you have a bad attitude about your new lifestyle, your body will always be listening, and you won't be able to stick to it! I often tell my clients, "Your body is listening to everything you say! Be careful what you think and say around it!" Time for an attitude check.

Secret #13: Manage your stress!

"Therefore do not worry about tomorrow, for tomorrow will worry about itself. Each day has enough trouble of its own."

—MATTHEW 6:34

Who isn't stressed these days? Everyone, especially women, has one too many things going on. Most women tend to take on not only all their own problems, but also everyone else's. Stress piles up on you and can wreak havoc on your health, your vitality, and your progress toward becoming a fit and empowered female. When your body is under excessive stress, you produce a hormone called cortisol, which is secreted by your adrenal glands. This hormone was meant to be secreted in fight-or-flight situations. For example, your body would churn out cortisol when you got scared because an animal was chasing you, and then you would run away and go sit in your cave and have what I call cortisol reduction time, when your adrenals would reboot for the next stressful event. Unfortunately, these days most women don't get much cortisol reduction time. Instead, their bodies are secreting cortisol 24/7, and as the day goes on, the stress increases and the cortisol keeps rising. When your stress and therefore your cortisol are high, your body is in a panicked state of survival. The last thing it's worried about is burning some fat or recovering from a workout.

Secret #14: Put an end to body bashing, and instead celebrate your strengths!

Women are so good at finding their own flaws but very rarely stop and enjoy what they love about their bodies. This is one difference between men and women.

Put an end to body bashing. Body bashers are very common among the female population. Women are constantly self-deprecating and bashing their own bodies. Be careful you don't join in with the bashing to try to make someone else feel better by

Battle of the Bulge

High stress = high belly fat! If your cortisol is chronically high, you may notice your amount of belly fat going up. Consistently, I see that when clients are under excessive stress and are letting it get the best of them, their belly fat increases. This has also been shown in research; a recent study revealed that women with high cortisol levels due to stress had an increase in their abdominal body fat. A fat belly is only going to make you more stressed! Be sure to include cortisol reduction time as part of your plan and don't let your tub overflow. And by the way, you can't take a pill to reduce cortisol effectively long term.

Fit Female Visual Tool

I share this analogy with my clients to help them manage stress. I first heard it from Paul Chek, who talked about it in relation to physiological load, which in the fit female world is stress. All of us have a tub that we fill with our stressful events. Some of us have huge tubs and can handle a lot of stress without it affecting us too much. Other people have smaller tubs and can't handle much at all, and the smallest obstacle in their life can overflow their small tub. Each stress is pouring into the tub from a faucet. Each type of stress has its own faucet. You may have one faucet pouring into your tub that is financial stress, another one that is relationship stress, another that's family stress, and another that's career stress. Identify all your faucets. What do you have flowing into your tub of stress? Some of these faucets may only be trickling in, while others are on full blast, quickly filling up your tub. The problems come when your tub gets full and starts to overflow. This is when you have symptoms of stress—you may develop anxiety or depression, or you may get sick. Everyone has a different response. But when your tub is overflowing, your body is not burning fat and building muscle— big problem. Instead, it is in a state of panic and will hold on to fat. Actually, when women are under extra stress and their tub is full, they carry more body fat on their bellies. There is no way you will get a six-pack if your tub is full of stress.

So, now that you're picturing your tub of stress with each of your faucets pouring into it and it is overflowing, what can you do to manage this?

1. Can you turn down or turn off any of the faucets? Can you hand off something that is stressing you out to someone else or not deal with it for the time being, until some of your other faucets are turned down? Decrease the amount of stress coming in if you can. If you absolutely cannot reduce the amount of stress, try prioritizing what can be dealt with right away.

2. Start putting drains in the bottom of your tub. Drains are actions you can take to destress. This includes cortisol reduction time, which is basically downtime to let your adrenals relax. Exercise can also be an outflow, as long as it's in the right amounts. Taking care of yourself, eating right, and getting enough sleep are all drains that will help you deal with the stress coming in. Start to think about ways you can drain some of the stress.

Use this visual and work on keeping your tub from overflowing, by keeping everything in perspective and not taking on too much. This will keep your body healthy, keep cortisol levels normal, and keep your body burning fat and building muscle so you can get your fit body. Fit females are in balance in every aspect of their lives and know how to handle and manage stress.

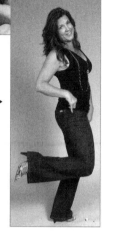

▲
Cheryl before

Cheryl lost 12 pounds of fat and dropped a clothing size **▶**

FIT FEMALE *Real Life Story*

My struggle with weight has always been intertwined with life's stresses and battling depression. A few months ago, I believed my world was racing out of control, and I found myself once again entering a dark place. While I was trying to swim to the surface without the help of a doctor or drug, the Fit Female Challenge was announced at Rachel's gym. It could be just the tool I needed to help turn things around on my own. When I decided to be a part of the challenge, I had set goals to lose fat, like all the other women. However, it turns out that an additional goal I made, to *gain* mental strength and happiness, became the real winner.

I started the challenge strong. I was determined to succeed, but when the results were slow to come, my focus began to slip, and I became frustrated. It was after a heart-to-heart with Rachel that I learned about how chronic stress produces cortisol in the body, which, in turn, contributes to the storage of body fat. So, not only was the stress affecting me mentally, it was also hurting me physically. The physical damage possible was made apparent again when I made a trip to urgent care, only to find out that the sharp pain in my diaphragm was gastritis, probably brought on by stress. I needed to make a point of consciously using outlets, or "drains," to help wash away and filter out the negative thoughts and energy. My daily workouts have been, and will always be, my strongest drains. For almost 25 years, exercise has been a constant in my life. No matter the number on the scale, I have never thought to stop. Lifting weights had begun to improve my muscle definition and tone; and while interval training strengthened my heart, it was also empowering me and giving me a boost of energy. Exercise has done as much for my brain as it has for my body. I just needed to stop, take a breath, and remember that.

My world was becoming brighter. I was once again finding joy in my day; and after a couple of months, I switched up my training schedule and started working out with a group of fit females early in the morning 4 days a week. Who knew that early mornings and exercise companions could make the journey so much more fun! My fat loss was only a quarter of what I was working toward. However, right now in my life, the clarity, joy, and gratitude I have gained back mean so much more. I will master the art of being 90 percent compliant with my nutrition, so that I can reach my personal goal of a healthy body fat percentage. I am not in a hurry, but I will continue to train, grow stronger, and enjoy the process! ✦

making a negative comment about your body. This is usually our instinct. Having a poor body image can be very contagious. If you have friends who are constantly ragging on how jiggly their thighs are or grabbing their pooch and drawing attention to their flaws, it's tempting to point out your own least favorite parts and join in on the negative talk. Instead, simply stop the nonsense: Tell them you think they look fabulous, and be genuine when you say it, then quickly change the subject. Put an end to the body bashing once and for all.

"Never dull your shine for somebody else."

—TYRA BANKS

Speaking of compliments, I have also noticed that body bashing is also very common when a woman receives a compliment on her body. A true fit female knows how to take a compliment and say thank you instead of replying with a potshot at herself, pointing out her flaws. "Who, me? What are you talking about? Forget it! I'm huge! Look at my muffin top!" Learn to say, "Thank you very much! I feel great!" and accept the compliment. As your body is changing, you'll receive more and more compliments, so be ready to respond to them. Remember, you are inspiring other people. As soon as you turn a compliment into a criticism, you have just sucked the inspiration right out of that person.

Think about what you love about your body and celebrate it! Instead of standing in front of the mirror and looking for your flaws, look in the mirror for your strengths. This is a a very important breakthrough. A true fit female looks in the mirror and is proud of who she is. One of my clients was constantly pointing out her flaws: "My arms are so big. I hate my stomach. . . . " I knew I had to stop this or she would never be successful. I asked her, "What do you love about your body?" After thinking for a long time, she responded, "My eyes." Perfect! So we focused on how gorgeous her eyes were when she looked in the mirror, and as her body was changing, we celebrated other areas that she was starting to like also, until eventually she liked her eyes and her legs. Then she liked her eyes, her legs, and her shoulders.

"We probably wouldn't worry about what people think of us if we could know how seldom they do."

—OLIN MILLER

Secret #15: Don't rely on willpower. Have strategies.

My good friend Valerie Waters, trainer to one of my favorite fit females, Jennifer Garner, said that strategies are a key part of her clients' success. She said, "Strategy trumps willpower. Studies show that willpower is actually in limited supply—meaning, resist the cookie now; it might be hard to resist it later. It truly is more important to build in good strategies."

Having strategies is absolutely one of the secrets of being fit and fabulous. I know for myself, one of my strategies is not to have anything in my house that is a trigger food. For me, this includes ice cream, cookies, or chocolate. If any of these foods are in my house, they will call my name and will eventually get eaten. I know I don't have the willpower to have these foods in my house. I never could understand people who say, "I can bake chocolate chip cookies and have them in my house and not touch one of them." What?! No way! If I am baking chocolate chip cookies, then I am planning to have a splurge, because I'll also be eating chocolate chip cookies! A key fit strategy is to keep healthy snacks in your house and not test your willpower by having junk food around. It will get eaten eventually.

There are lots of other strategies that can help keep you from relying on willpower alone. For instance, if you find yourself always blowing your diet at a certain time of day, you need to come up with a strategy for that time of day, such as having some almonds in your purse to snack on, or making sure you eat enough earlier in the day, or carrying an ice chest with you with a plan for exactly what you'll use to fuel your body, so it isn't left to chance. Never leave your fit body to chance—it won't happen by accident. If you always give in when you go out to dinner, you need to have a strategy, which might be that you'll go out to dinner no more than once a week. Use the strategies from the nutrition chapter in this book and all the tools I give you to get through your tough times and have success. Don't count on willpower. Figure out strategies that will work for you.

CLOTHING

What you wear in the gym is very important. Usually women start their journey wearing baggy T-shirts and sweats, but as they feel better about themselves, they celebrate their progress by showing off some skin or at least wearing tighter clothes. It is important to wear clothing that lets you see the shape of your body changing in the mirror when you work out. If you wear a big potato sack all the time, you can't see the changes that are happening. Get a tight pair of flattering pants and a tight shirt, and when you're ready, break out the sports bra or at least a tank top and show off your killer fit body. I always make my clients start to dress in tighter, more revealing clothes as they're changing. I believe it is extremely powerful in their transformation to becoming fit. Secret: Wearing a half top while you're working out will force you to keep your tummy tight for the whole workout, and you will see abs peeking through before you know it. Remember, you have to act as if you are a fit female to become one, so start dressing like one!

Secret #16: Stop rationalizing and making excuses!

"Rationalizations are generally convenient evasions of reality and are used as excuses for dishonest behavior, mistakes, and/or laziness."

—DAVE KEKICH

Spare me your excuses, sister! I work with clients daily and hear every excuse in the book. Everyone has an excuse or their own rationalization for why they can't lift more weight, eat healthier, or push their limits. And you will *always* be able to find one—*always!* Stop putting the blame elsewhere and take ownership of your body. There is always an excuse not to start today.

"When you make an excuse, you are only telling a lie to yourself."

—UNKNOWN

There is also no room for "kinda, sorta, maybe," meaning that if I ask you, "Are you following the Fit Female Credo, training program, and nutrition program?" you can only answer yes or no; you cannot answer "kinda" or "somewhat" or "I am, *but . . .*" or "I'm trying." These all mean your answer is NO. Anytime you use the word *try,* you may as well replace it with "I am giving myself an out because I am planning to fail." Don't expect to become a fit female if you're only "kinda, sorta, maybe trying" to follow the advice I've so painstakingly laid out in this book.

"Do . . . or do not. There is no 'try.'"

—JEDI MASTER YODA

Some of the most common excuses I hear for putting off taking action and becoming a fit female are listed below. If any of them

BE READY TO MAKE A BIG SACRIFICE IF YOU SMOKE

Apparently, some women still think smoking looks sexy. A report done in 2001 by the surgeon general showed that 22 percent of American women smoked. You cannot be a fit female and smoke cigarettes. Smoking goes against everything fit being stands for. A fit female is healthy, takes care of her body, and feels good about herself. There is nothing healthy about smoking. Research has linked smoking to the No. 1 killer of women, cardiovascular disease. Smoking is also linked to higher risks of numerous cancers, including lung cancer, which kills more women than breast cancer. And if that isn't enough, a study done on 132 pairs of twins showed that smoking can also cause a three- to fivefold increase in thyroid disease. Considering that the thyroid controls metabolism (a word you'll be hearing a lot throughout this book), we don't want to do anything to mess with the thyroid. And if getting cardiovascular disease, cancer, or thyroid disease isn't enough to scare you, don't forget that research has shown that smoking causes wrinkles by prematurely aging the skin. What good is having an amazing fit body if you're all wrinkly? If you smoke, it's time to quit. Picture who you want to become and rid yourself of the habits that will keep you from getting there. Put out the cigarette once and for all.

sound familiar, then it's time to stop making excuses.

✦ **"I don't have enough time!"**

This is the most common excuse and it drives me crazy! Ladies, here's a little secret: You don't *find* time—you *make* time!

"Until you value yourself, you won't value your time. Until you value your time, you will not do anything with it."

—M. SCOTT PECK

You will *never* suddenly have all this extra time to exercise and prepare your meals, and the good news is it probably doesn't take as much time as you think. But you have to decide you want this. You only get one shot at life, and as time goes by, days go by, and years go by, you do not get them back. That's it—one opportunity to make the best out of your given time. Are you setting time aside for yourself, or are you wasting it doing something else? Like maybe . . . coming up with excuses? Isn't it amazing how much time we have to rationalize and create excuses for ourselves?

You should think of time as being equal to life. Replace the word *time* with the word *life* from now on. When you don't have enough time, you don't have enough life to get in shape and reach your potential physically and mentally. Time = life. What do you want in your life? If it is to be a fit, confident, and empowered, then make the time.

Or decide that your life is not worth it. If you don't have time now in your life, then you'd better have time later to regret never reaching your potential physically and mentally. The pain of having regrets far outweighs taking the time now to plan your day and make fitness and eating right a priority in your life. Life is too short to not look and feel your absolute best every single day.

"The future is something which everyone reaches at the rate of 60 minutes an hour, whatever he does, whoever he is."

—C. S. LEWIS

When it comes to changing your body, it doesn't take as much time as you may think to get results. In fact, in many cases, less is more for those of you who are cardio queens. The program in this book will take three to six hours a week, total. Keep in mind, I have also had clients get amazing results doing two hours a week. If you really are limited, something is better than nothing, and if you make those two hours count and are doing effective workouts like the ones in this book, you will see results. The key to changing your body is consistently working toward your goal week after week. I'm sure you can spare an hour two to six times a week for exercise. Not having time is no longer an excuse. Make time to accomplish what you want in your life. Why not go through life feeling fit, confident, and empowered? You will never get back lost time. Stop making excuses. Simply ask yourself, "Is this the best use of my time right now to get me closer to my goal of becoming the fit and fabulous female I want to become?"

Take the time to plan out your day and make becoming fit a priority. Remember Secret #6— Be an early riser and get it done before anything else gets in your way. No more excuses, no more regrets. There is nothing to it but to do it.

Make time to become the fit, confident, empowered person you want to become. You're worth it, and you have the time. Really!

✦ **"I am destined to be fat. It's in my genes."**

I have no patience for this excuse, because I come from a family of people who all struggle with their weight, most of whom are obese. Yes, it is harder for me, because my body does like to store fat. If I didn't work out and watch what I eat, I would also be obese. I have to watch my diet pretty closely and push myself hard in the gym, but I would never use that as an excuse not to be the best I can be. Some people are skinny without trying, no matter what. Good for them. That doesn't mean you should just give in to your genetics and be fat and unsatisfied, never reaching your potential in life. It will take some work, but you can look and feel amazing no matter what your genetics are. Take it from me!

✦ **"I'm on my period, and I have cramps."**

I hear this one a lot. You will actually feel better if you exercise. I mean it. One of the reasons you feel down in the dumps at this time of the month is that your level of the brain chemical serotonin is low. Exercise boosts serotonin naturally and will make you feel better. Also, the movement will help to alleviate some of the symptoms and will make you feel better. Plus, it will keep you from sitting around having a pity party because you're bloated and on your period,

and I know what goes along with a pity party . . . chocolate. Get to the gym! Also, as your body is changing, your hormones should stabilize and reduce or eliminate menstrual cramps. There! You have something to look forward to. Read the chapter on hormones for some tips on getting through this time of the month still feeling fit and fabulous.

✦ **"Work is hectic. I have too much to do at work."**

This goes back to Secret #1—You have to make time. Work will always be there. Life is passing you by while you are busy working. You should take time for yourself every single day. Exercising will give you more energy at work, clear your head, and make you more productive. Work is not an acceptable excuse. Take an hour a day for yourself, no exceptions. If it means waking up an hour earlier, do it!

✦ **"Eating the same foods is so boring. I'm sick of chicken and vegetables."**

Sounds like whining. Eating does not, and should not, equal entertainment. First of all, you have a whole bunch of different foods on the grocery list in the nutrition chapter, so you can eat a large variety of foods. Get creative! And second, you need to enjoy fueling your body and how the healthy food makes you feel. Tune in to how great you feel when you're eating those "boring" foods. The feeling you get by being in shape should outweigh how boring the food is.

Keep a good attitude and pick out different stuff from the grocery list every week.

✦ **"I'm too tired."**

Have a strategy that you will always go to the gym and start your workout. Do one set of everything and see how you feel. If you're still exhausted and not into it, go home and get some R & R. You can still feel good that you did one set and come back and hit it hard in a day or two. But usually once you get started, the endorphins increase, the tiredness begins to fade, and you start feeling better. Believe me, I don't always want to work out, and I've been tired, but I have never regretted doing a workout. Keep in mind that as much as you may not feel like working out, once you're finished, you'll be glad you did, and you will never regret it.

✦ **"I walk. Isn't that enough?"**

No. It is not enough. What happened to our society that walking is now considered exercise? Walking is part of living an active lifestyle. You should walk when you can, but it is not the challenge that will transform your body. You have to put a challenge on your body that it's not used to in order to get it to change. Go for a walk as part of your relaxation.

✦ **"I'm too stressed!"**

When you are under a lot of stress, you actually need exercise even more. The right amount of exercise can be a drain in your tub to help you manage stress, relieve some of the tension, and boost your endorphins to make you feel good.

✦ **"My kids come first."**

I work with a lot of moms who are constantly taking care of everyone else. They wake up every day and make sure everyone else is taken care of and has what they need. Their children count on them every single day. It's hard for these women to stop and take an hour out of their day to take care of themselves and not someone else. But, as a mother, if you don't take care of yourself, you are actually being selfish. Don't you owe it to your kids and family to be the best you can be, feeling full of energy, feeling good about yourself, and being a healthy role model for your children to look up to? If you, as the mom everyone depends on, break down . . . then what? You have to take care of yourself first so you can take care of everyone else. This is not an excuse in my book, but all the more reason why you *have* to make exercise and eating right a priority.

✦ **"I fit in my clothes and don't need to exercise. I feel good enough."**

Is life about just getting by, settling for "good enough"? No, it's about living life to the fullest, feeling and looking your absolute best, and having fulfilling relationships and experiences that are all a part of being the best you can be, not just "good enough." Life is not about just getting by. Don't settle for "good enough."

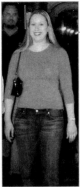

FIT FEMALE *Real Life Story*

Since becoming a fit female, I have become much more aware of my diet. I realize now that when I do eat junk food, it makes me feel tired and unhealthy. Working out

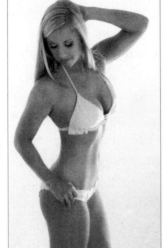

▲
Gerry in her size 12s before she lost 30 pounds of fat.

Gerry is fabulous as a size 4. ▶

in the morning motivates me to eat healthily and make better choices throughout the rest of the day. I also don't feel as guilty if I do treat myself to a dessert, because I know that I can just work harder in the gym the next day.

Before becoming a fit female, I was unhappy in many of the clothes that I put on. I was self-conscious about my arms, so I would avoid sleeveless shirts or tank tops. I also avoided tight shirts that would cling to my stomach. I tried to dress in a way that would hide my flaws, but then I would see pictures and realize I wasn't fooling anyone.

Now, it's like I have an entirely new wardrobe. Things that I would try on before and just put straight back on the hanger fit me differently now. My jeans are all too big now, so I finally bought a new pair. I also gave away all my old jeans as a way of motivating myself to stay fit and never go back to my old size.

Today, I feel stronger and more defined. Each week I'm surprised by the muscle definition that I'm seeing. I didn't think my body was capable of being this lean, and it feels good. I feel like it's still me, but in a new and improved package. I'm feeling much more confident all around, making me walk a little taller and prouder.

Even if I'm stressed about school or work, it's nice not to add "I feel fat" to my list of stresses. I know that when I'm feeling a little depressed or down, feeling overweight or out of shape adds to that in a big way. It's a huge relief to feel good about my body physically, which is a hard thing to change. I can honestly say that completing the Fit Female Challenge has changed how I live my life . . . and I will never go back!

I know that in order to be happy, I need to be a fit female.

When I am fit, I feel fabulous! ✦

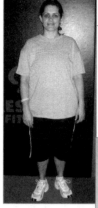

▲
**Cheralyn
before**

**Cheralyn lost
40 pounds
of fat and
8 clothing
sizes.** ▶

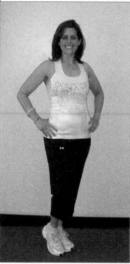

FIT FEMALE *Real Life Story*

I love how I feel! I've been living for years with the excuse,"It's not my time—
when my kids grow up I'll have time to focus on myself." But then I realized
that my kids were getting ripped off just as much as I
was. There's no way I can be the best that my kids
deserve when I am not at my best. My excuse wasn't
working anymore and it was time to make some
changes. I sheepishly began my first workout program at Results and it was so pathetic I couldn't even
do 6 lunges in a row. Incorporating the nutrition plan
seemed daunting and finding time to work out was a
constant struggle. It seemed like there was always a
good reason why "today" wasn't a good day. But
that's just it—it's all about today. It has to be today.
Today is the day I need to think about my health, my
fitness, my intentions. Pretty soon "tomorrow" will be
"today," so I had to start thinking of what I was doing
to meet my goals, every single day. I committed myself to following the plan 100%. I was determined to start working out regularly and give my best effort every time and I always ended with
a recovery shake—the best part of my day! The incredible thing is I couldn't believe how quickly
the changes occurred. Within a few weeks I felt stronger, I had more energy, and I could see my
body changing. Soon I wasn't even thinking of looking for excuses anymore—I wanted to be in
the gym! 6 months later the clothes I used to hide in my closet because they were too tight have
been thrown out because they are too big. I am doing exercises I never dreamed of and loving it,
and the nutrition plan is my new comfort zone because I know every day that I am doing my
body good and the guesswork is gone. Even my aching joints and headaches are no longer a
problem. I find myself smiling as I walk into the gym and smiling even bigger on the way out. I
am more anxious to be out and about, and I love shopping again! My kids tell me I'm strong and
they love how much I am willing to do with them. Even after 4 kids and heading towards 40, I
really don't know when I've ever felt better. It's totally worth it and I can't wait to see where I am
in another 6 months!"—Cheralyn Goekeritz ✦

Chapter 2

From Frumpy and Frowny to Fit and Fabulous

Maybe you have hit your all-time low mentally and physically, are wearing your frumpy fat clothes, and have lost all hope that you'll ever get into your skinny jeans again. Or maybe you've never even owned a pair of skinny jeans and have always wondered what it would be like to feel good about your body. You have a hard time picturing yourself as anything other than "bigger" or the "fat friend." You constantly beat yourself up about being fat and try on 20 different outfits every time you get dressed, because you hate the way everything looks. This outfit makes your butt look even fatter. That one shows your cellulite, and you can't wear that one because your belly flab is hanging over. You won't be caught dead in shorts, wearing a tank top, flaunting your stuff in a bathing suit, or, God forbid, actually getting naked. No way! Or maybe you are in okay shape and feel all right in clothes but are ready to take your body to the next level. Maybe what you've been doing up until this point has stopped working, and you're looking for something different to finally reach your ultimate body.

Keep in mind that even if you have failed at losing weight and keeping it off in the past, there is hope. The National Weight Control Registry is conducting an ongoing study following more than 5,000 men and women who have lost an average of 66 pounds or more and kept it off for at least five years. Among the participants, 91 percent had tried and failed in the past. So don't lose hope if nothing else has worked for you. Instead, realize that you are actually even closer to figuring it out for yourself.

Wherever you are, I have been there. I also have clients who have been there. Throughout this book, I will share my stories and those of my clients, and I guarantee within these pages you will connect, be inspired, and find your switch to transform your life and become a fit female. While I wrote this book, I not only reflected on my own experiences but also reexamined the interactions I have daily with the women I coach in the gym. At our gym, with the help of my staff, we have worked with more than a thousand women in the over nine years we've been open, and I have learned something from every single one of them and continue to learn from them. The accumulation of my experience with my own body and working with more than a thousand women to reach their potential physically and mentally is what inspires the contents of this book. Real results, achieved with real people, and sharing what really works.

Before I made the breakthrough and figured out what works for me, I struggled with my weight and body image my entire life. I grew up in a very close, loving family who just happened to love food as much as we loved each other. Whether it was a time to celebrate, a stressful time, a good day, or a bad day, we needed to have food surrounding us. Supposedly, everything was always better with food. My entire family struggles with their weight and still, to this day, uses food when stress arises. I quickly learned to check out from a stressful day by bingeing on junk food. Food became my drug of choice. I have been at the lowest of lows with my body image, have been depressed, have struggled with binge eating and bulimia, and at one point felt like I would never be in control of my relationship with food or feel good about my body. I have struggled with starvation diets, counting calories, doing endless aerobics classes, and always trying to achieve the look of a fit female.

As I said earlier, wherever you are right now, I've been there. I know exactly how you feel. I haven't always felt fit and fabulous. This is not your typical book written by a fitness guru who has always been in shape and has no idea what it feels like to be in your shoes. Along with being in your shoes, I've also been seeking information from every resource—earning a degree in physiology and learning everything I could about the human body, reading and interpreting the research, studying the experts in the industry and asking questions, and being on a pursuit to be the best at helping women reach their potential physically and mentally.

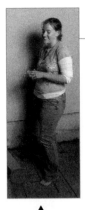

▲

Lisa before covering up her frumpiness, in her size 12s.

Lisa as a fit female ▶ **showing off her fabulousness as a size 6.**

FIT FEMALE *Real Life Story*

I had never been in a gym. The only exercise I had done was in PE in school, and I played softball. That was it. I had lost weight before by following the Weight

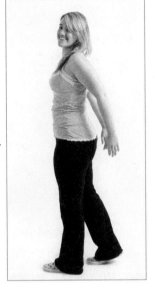

Watchers points system, but I had never really exercised to get the weight off. Following the Weight Watchers plan, I always felt like I never had many points to use, and once I had reached my goal, I knew I was skinny, but I always felt as if I was skinny fat— meaning my body looked like a smaller version of the same flabby body. [For more on skinny fat, see page 29.]

Plus, I eventually gained back almost all the weight I had lost, so I guess it didn't really work long term.

One day I was hanging out with friends, and I was starting to feel like the "fat friend." You know, that one girl in the group of skinny girls who is really nice but never gets a date. Then I decided that I didn't want to be the fat friend anymore. I set up some goals, and I lost about 10 pounds over 12 weeks by following a strength-training program similar to the one in this book, designed for me at Rachel's gym, Results Fitness. After that, I was feeling good, and I was hooked. I kept losing weight and stuck with what I was doing.

Then Rachel challenged me to dial it in even more with my nutrition. At first I was hesitant about changing my diet. Going through Weight Watchers, I had to change my diet, and while I didn't change it drastically, it was enough to make me not want to do it again for any diet. In the end, I decided that I would challenge myself to dial my nutrition in and see how far I got.

I was so surprised to find that the Fit Female Nutrition Rules are really easy to follow, and once they become a habit, there is no going back. It really is easy and is now a part of my lifestyle. I pack my snacks every day and plan out my meals.

I've lost 20 pounds of fat and have gone down three clothing sizes! I'm feeling fit and fabulous. Now, instead of being the fat friend, I'm the hot, confident friend! ✦

Besides that, I have been at every extreme when it comes to body composition. It's like Goldilocks and the Three Bears. I've tried every porridge, I've tried every kind of body on for size, and I've figured out the right fit for me. Don't believe me? Check this out!

AEROBICS INSTRUCTOR, RINKY-DINK PINK DUMBBELL BODY (23 TO 25% BODY FAT)

I was teaching 10 to 12 aerobics classes a week. That's 10-plus hours of aerobics a week. I also lifted light dumbbells (yes, they were probably pink) for lots of repetitions and *never* lifted any weights with my legs, because they were already big and I didn't want them to get any bigger. Once in a while I would do the inner- and outer-thigh machine to tone my inner thighs. This was strange logic, now that I look back—why did I think the weights were going to make my upper body look defined and small, but for some reason using weights with my lower body would bulk them up? And what was my deal with the inner- and outer-thigh machine—why did I think that would make my inner and outer thighs smaller somehow? None of it worked anyway. I was in good shape, but I had aerobics instructor chunky thigh syndrome, a term first coined by Charles Poliquin. *Aerobics instructor chunky thigh syndrome* is a phrase I've heard used by more than one person in the fitness industry, but it

AEROBICS INSTRUCTOR CHUNKY THIGH SYNDROME:

A phenomenon experienced by an aerobics instructor who teaches at least six to 10 classes a week (for some, up to three hours a day) and whose body has completely adapted to aerobic exercise, to the point where it stores fat more efficiently than it burns fat. She has turned her body into a highly efficient fat-storing machine instead of a fat-burning machine. Typically, the fat tends to be stored disproportionately in the lower body. The average aerobics instructor has about 22 percent to 24 percent body fat (a healthy range but not that of a fit female), and all the chub is on her butt and thighs.

does not seem to have made it out into the general public.

As for myself, I tend to carry more fat on my lower body regardless. However, doing 10 or more aerobics classes a week and staying away from the heavy weights so I didn't get big and bulky made my lower body even chunkier. I had created the perfect environment for my lower body to store fat by not building any muscle and by doing a ton of aerobics so it would adapt enough to become efficient at storing fat. I never wore shorts, because I hated my legs. It wasn't until I started to lift weights—and I'm talking *real* weights, not rinky-dink pink ones—and cut back on the aerobics that I really saw my body change. That was when I started to look like the fit female I had always wanted to be.

I tried out this "aerobics doesn't work for fat loss" theory again later down the road, when I trained for an Ironman Triathlon and swam, biked, and ran my way to completing a 2.4-mile swim, a 112-mile bike ride, and a marathon, all in one day. I was doing 20 to 30 hours of aerobic exercise a week to train for it. My findings were consistent: Aerobics doesn't work for fat loss. And training for the Ironman proved that doing even more of it wasn't the answer, either. More about this in Chapter 3, Change Your Paradigms, Change Your Body.

Skinny fat: A body type that I have never had myself, but may describe you, is skinny fat. Women who are skinny fat are slender and wear a small clothing size, but they have never worked out and have no muscle tone or definition. If you grabbed their arm, it would feel like mush with a bone in the middle. They look good in clothes, but they usually have a flat butt with no shape, because they have no muscle. The average person looking at a skinny fat woman would not understand how she could be unhappy with her body, but most of these women really aren't happy, because deep down they know they are actually not in shape, even though they appear skinny. They have a very high percentage of fat as a proportion of their total weight. I've had many skinny fat women as clients, and they all want to change their bodies to be firm and have definition. So, if you are skinny fat, this program will also work for you to turn you into a fit female.

You have experienced this body if you have been a cardio queen and have made aerobics your priority when it comes to working out. You may have lost weight by dieting and doing excessive cardio, but you looked the same, just smaller, or your body adapted and you never got to where you wanted to be.

EXTREMELY LEAN AND RIPPED FITNESS COMPETITOR BODY (10 TO 12% BODY FAT)

Soon after I started lifting "real" weights and cutting back on my aerobics, I became hooked on the changes my body was making and decided to take it to the next level and compete in fitness. I remember lifting heavier and heavier weights as my body was getting smaller and smaller. It was amazing. I was really figuring out how to use weight training to transform my body. I was not doing aerobics at all, and with every workout, I would push myself to lift heavier and challenge my body. This is when I first lifted 50-pound dumbbells doing an incline chest press. I also used 45-pound dumbbells (one in each hand) while doing lunges, and I did my first chinup! I was hooked! I was no longer afraid to lift heavy with my lower body, because I could see that I was finally getting my legs to look the way I wanted them to. The more I lifted, the smaller, leaner, and more defined I became. I felt confident about the way I looked.

I took a good thing to the extreme. I had to

have obsessive discipline with my diet to get down below 15 percent body fat to compete. I learned that my body doesn't like to get that lean. Some women have body types that can stay around 13 to 15 percent body fat year round, but not me. It took extreme measures to trick my body to get down to that level. I also had to add extra workout sessions leading up to the contest to trim every ounce of fat.

During this time, diet and exercise consumed my life. They had to in order for me to get this lean for a fitness competition, what would be called "ripped" in the fitness world.

This was not something I could maintain long term. It took extreme discipline, with no room for a splurge. I didn't feel good this lean. I *looked* good but didn't feel good. I have to work hard not to get fat (you'll see what I mean in my next photo), so getting this lean was very difficult for me. I loved competing and getting onstage and challenging myself to accomplish that goal, but there was no way I could maintain that body forever. I was shredded, ripped, whatever adjective you want to use, but I was not living life to the fullest—I was tired, depleted, hungry, deprived, and unhappy. This was not my best body, because I did not feel optimal. I'm not saying I wouldn't ever push my body to these limits again, but knowing what I know now, I would handle the post-competition season differently. Now I realize I could never expect myself to maintain that body. When I work with fitness and figure

RIPPED:

Ripped is when you burn off every ounce of fat to the point that you start to see the contours of every muscle and even veins. It is also called "shredded" in the fitness world. It is beyond being defined and toned. The difference between losing fat and getting ripped is a matter of the degree of fat you lose. Being a fit female, you do not want to be ripped. This is taking a good thing too far.

competitors—and I work with quite a few—I always tell them, "You are achieving a look and a body fat level that will peak for one night. You will not be able to maintain it. It is not a healthy body fat level." I wish I had known this back when I was a fitness competitor. Instead, I started to beat myself up and get into a very negative mindset that spiraled out of control.

If you have done any kind of extreme diet and workout plan in which you were superfocused, had tunnel vision, and put everything else in your life on hold, you have also been at a point where you may have thought you'd achieved the body you wanted. It's important to know that staying there is nearly impossible when you get back to normal. You shouldn't have to suffer, be deprived, and be completely consumed by your diet and exercise to achieve your fit female body. That is not what it's about. You have to learn to get the body you want and still live life to the fullest, enjoying every moment of every day.

BUSTING-OUT-OF-MY-FAT-CLOTHES BODY (29%+ BODY FAT)

After being so disciplined with my diet and exercise and seeing what my body could look like at an extreme level, I developed a very destructive mindset, because my body would not maintain the fitness competitor leanness that had become the new ideal in my head. The pendulum began to swing back in the other direction. I had since moved back in with my family and had some stress in my life. And, if you remember what I said earlier, where my family is, food is! And what better way to deal with stress than with food? My old habits of bingeing came right back. I let myself go and got up to the heaviest I had ever been—40 pounds heavier than I am today and probably 29 to 30 percent body fat. This didn't last too long, as I refused to buy a bigger size when I was busting out of my fat clothes. I think I was up to a size 14 or 16 at this point. I knew I had to take action.

I realized that this was where my body would continue going if I paid no attention to what I ate and didn't exercise. If I didn't consciously work at it, I would be obese. I did not feel good and hated the way I looked in clothes. I was exactly like the example I was talking about earlier, trying on 10 different outfits before just giving up. I was not fat and happy. I was fat and unhappy. I decided I would never let myself get to this point again.

If this is where you are, I have been there and know how you feel. Nothing fits, you're squishy all over, and you're insecure about your body. You have to decide that you will never let this happen again. Take action today to move away from it. You are in control of your body.

FIT FEMALE BODY (18 TO 20% BODY FAT)

Finally, the porridge that is "just right." I don't have to do hours and hours of exercise. I can enjoy an occasional splurge of a glass of wine or maybe dessert and not feel guilty. I work out a reasonable four to six days a week for up to an hour each session. I do have to push myself in the gym and make every workout count, challenge my body consistently, and pay attention to what I eat, but I don't obsess about anything. I fuel my body with healthy foods, have energy and vitality to enjoy life, and feel confident about the way I look. I love working out, but my workouts don't consume my life. Being a fit female is about living life to the fullest, having time and energy for your friends and family, and feeling good because you have your best body. I can grab any outfit out of my closet, throw it on, and head out feeling good about myself. I enjoy going shopping for clothes, even bathing suit shopping. Seriously,

I do. I feel confident in my own body and am able to wear anything I want and feel good about myself, even wearing . . . nothing at all.

THIS *IS* JUST US GIRLS TALKING, RIGHT?

Yes, ladies, we can admit it. Part of being a fit female is feeling sexy again and feeling confident to take your clothes off with the lights on. After all, one reason women work out and watch what they eat is to look and feel better in *and* out of clothes. You don't want to just look good in clothes. You want to be able to run around your house in boy short panties and a tank top feeling confident about how you look. We all want to be that girl—confident, secure about her body! When you feel good enough to take your clothes off with the lights on and wear sexy clothes more often, you'll be ready to enjoy your new body with a romp in the bedroom with your significant other more often, too, leading to more fulfilling relationships. More than once, I've had clients' husbands thank me and tell me that we should be marriage counselors. I'm not kidding. Feeling sexy and empowered and enjoying your new body has far-reaching benefits!

"Sex appeal is 50 percent what you've got and 50 percent what people think you've got."

—SOPHIA LOREN

Being healthy is nice, and being able to lift your groceries and function better is great, but bottom line, you want to feel hot and be able to wear anything. You want to be the girl the other women in the room are calling a B-I-T-C-H because she looks so good. Remember, BITCH stands for Be Inspiring, Totally Confident, and Hot! You want to be the girl every woman wants to *be* and every man wants to *be with*. You know—the girl you may have been jealous of, the one you and your girlfriends were whispering about, or maybe you were just telling each other, *"That* is what I want to look like." Why can't *that* be you?

"There are no good girls gone wrong, just bad girls found out."

—MAE WEST

So, as I said before, wherever you are mentally and physically, I've been there. Everybody is different and will look different in their best body. My best fit female body may be very different from yours. Some women can maintain a fitness competitor lean body much more easily than I could. Most women I've seen feel good about themselves and have the feeling of being a fit female at about 18 to 20 percent body fat. I like to talk in body fat and clothing size because the number on the scale will change as you gain muscle and isn't a good indicator of where you are. Your weight is not the whole picture and tells you only a piece of the puzzle.

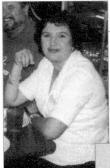

▲
**Donna
before**

**Donna as a
fit female,** ▶
**She lost
39 pounds
of fat and
4 clothing
sizes.**

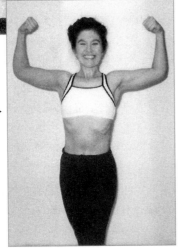

FIT FEMALE *Real Life Story*

A few weeks after my 38th birthday, I decided I didn't like the way I
looked. This wasn't your typical "Gee, I don't like the way I look today."
This was more of an overwhelming "Gee, I
don't like the way I look today or *any* day!" My
self-esteem was at an all-time low. The thought
of going to dinner and a movie sent me into a
tailspin, because I hated the way I looked in my
clothes. Even worse, I hated the way I looked
and felt *without* my clothes. I thought to
myself, "If I started getting in shape now, then
maybe, just maybe I'll have the body I've
always wanted by the time I'm 40." So I began
training on March 16, 2000. My goal was to
lose 25 pounds of fat before Memorial Day—
less than 11 weeks away.

As I began to lose weight and gain muscle,
the first thing I noticed, or should I say the first thing my husband noticed, was that my self-
esteem was on the rise. I began wearing tighter clothes and struttin' around the house like I was
"all that and a bag of chips." If you're not familiar with this '90s expression, it means a really hot
girl who's got it going on, who's all that and more . . . and that's exactly how I felt. It was amazing. I couldn't remember the last time I'd felt this way, or if I ever had.

I not only achieved my goal of losing 25 pounds of fat before Memorial Day, I exceeded my
goal—and I did it in just 8 weeks! Ultimately, I lost 39 pounds of fat and gained 10 pounds of lean,
toned muscle, and my body fat has gone from 36 percent to 17 percent. I'm not suggesting it was
easy—but it's a whole lot easier than you might think. I lifted weights two days a week on my lunch
break and did not have to do any boring cardio. I can honestly say I never really believed I would
truly be in the best condition of my life at age 40! ✦

FIT FEMALE *Real Life Story*

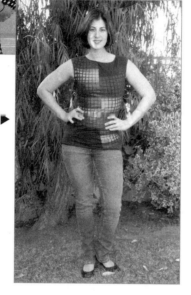

▲
Tania before

Tania as a fit female. She lost 30 pounds of fat and 3 clothing sizes. ►

I must say that two back-to-back pregnancies took a toll on my body. Before I got pregnant the first time, I weighed 140 pounds at 5 feet 6 inches. With my first baby, I gained close to 35 pounds, taking all the precautions necessary. Four months after the delivery, and at 153 pounds, I got pregnant again. This time I gained 43 pounds, even with a more cautious diet and pregnancy yoga classes. By the time of delivery, I weighed 196 pounds.

I was really bothered by my weight, and I knew the only way I would be light on my feet again and as energetic as before was to commit to an exercise program and a diet adjustment. Oh yeah! Did I mention I wanted results that were quick and long lasting?

Turns out, strength training, meaning weight lifting and resistance training, has proven itself to be the answer.

Less than a year after starting my strength-training program, I weighed 140 pounds again. But wait . . . I got more than just weight loss. My body is strong; I have active muscles I have never had before in all parts of my body. My flexibility has improved, and my chronic knee pain is hardly ever a problem anymore. My metabolism has increased, and so has my food intake. Of course, I'm not noshing on cookies and chocolate all the time, but I haven't really eliminated them from my diet, either. Instead, I enjoy them in moderation. As I continue every week in my resistance-training program, I feel stronger and leaner.

Overall, my body withstood a transformation from fat to fat loss to muscle formation. This program has helped me create a healthy body and mind. The best part: I am a really energetic and proud mommy of two-year-old and one-year-old boys. ✦

You have to figure out what your best body is, where you look and feel absolutely amazing. Don't focus on a number, but on a feeling, one of confidence and empowerment! Most women are too focused on a magic number and forget to tune in to how they *feel* and how they look in their clothes. One of my clients said to me recently, "When you get to your best body and feel confident and sexy, the feeling is like a high you never want to come off of, so it's easy to keep. Once you feel that high, you'll never let it go!" I can't wait for you to experience the same feeling. And once you do, you'll be hooked.

Over 12 years ago, I hit rock bottom and really went on a quest once and for all to figure out this body image thing and gain control over my body. Since then, I've been able to test my principles when life throws obstacles my way. I like to think of our gym as our own personal laboratory where we can figure out exactly what works and what doesn't while our clients give us constant feedback. We're always fine-tuning our strat-egies for achieving the best results possible. We track every single workout and the progress our clients make. We now have over nine years of data on working with women whose No. 1 goal is to become a fit female—some of whom you've already met, and even more to come. You will connect with a story, be inspired by a picture, or be motivated by a refreshing new way to approach your workouts and nutrition.

Up until now, what I know and have learned from experience with myself and my clients has been shared only with members of our gym. My hope is that through this book I can reach out to millions of women who are looking for something different, who want to make a breakthrough, and who are ready to commit. I want to help you find your inner strength and give you the same feeling I have and my clients have of being confident, empowered, and sexy! I will be with you throughout this book and throughout your entire journey. Instead of being frumpy and frowny, you will be fit and fabulous!

Chapter 3

Change Your Paradigms, Change Your Body

What do your workouts currently consist of? Are you a cardio queen, or do you avoid the gym altogether? Maybe your workouts consist of a recommended hour of cardio a day, and sometimes you'll do a couple of aerobics classes in a row, or you'll spend hours on the treadmill going nowhere. Maybe you stick to the rinky-dink, tiny weights and barely break a sweat, afraid to actually challenge yourself because you're afraid you'll sprout big, bulky muscles or become "too masculine." More likely, you don't want to actually see any results! You might hit the abductor, adductor, and butt blaster every once in a while and maybe pick up some light weights for a lot of repetitions, because again, you're afraid spontaneous muscles might pop up, so you don't want to lift too heavy. If you don't have time to fit everything in, you skip your weights completely and just do your cardio workout. After all, it burns the most calories . . . you think. You watch what you eat and stick to low-fat foods while keeping your calories low, starving your muscles of enough protein so, once again, they don't get too big and bulky.

All this and I bet you are completely frustrated, because your body isn't changing and you don't look anything like a fit female. Or maybe you don't work out at all, because in the past you've become frustrated after not having any success doing all of the above, so you gave up. I'm sure there are also some of you who have never worked out, because doing all of the above is not appealing to you at all, and you decided that if that's what's necessary, forget it!

So how do you get to look like a fit female?

What does she know that you don't know?

First of all, a fit female is not afraid of challenging herself in the gym. She knows the only way to change her body is to put demands on it that are outside of her comfort zone. She looks toned and defined because she is strong and has muscle, the very thing you may fear you'll build. Her strength training is her No. 1 priority because she knows it gives her the defined look she wants and boosts her metabolism. She doesn't spend more than an hour in the gym at a time, and she pushes herself during that hour. She'll burn more calories in the 24 to 48 hours following her workout because of the demands she has put on her body and the intensity at which she trains. She takes her workout seriously, keeping track of her progress by writing down the weights she lifted and how she felt. She has a plan for her workout and goes to the gym with a strength-training program that she changes every few weeks to keep her body from adapting. She also knows that she shouldn't change the program too often, or she won't know if she's making progress. She loves the feeling of being strong and fit and challenging herself in the gym, whether it's with dumbbells, chinups, pushups, or a barbell. In her world, muscle and strength are good things. She knows that she will never look like a man because she is not a man and does not have the biological makeup to look like one. Instead, the stronger and more fit she gets, the more defined and sculpted her body will be and the higher her metabolism will be. She does not focus on the scale, but instead on how her clothes fit, how she feels, and how she looks. She fuels her body with lots of good food and eats every couple of hours, constantly feeding her metabolism. She does not deprive herself and knows how to fit in a splurge if she wants one without wreaking havoc on her body composition.

If you want toned arms, you have to lift enough weight to actually build muscle. That tone is actually muscle that was built with weights heavy enough to be challenging. Remember, you have to put a demand on your body beyond what it's used to in order for it to change. By really lifting weights and challenging your muscles, you will increase your lean mass, which is what really burns fat. Lean mass is what gives you the capacity to burn more fat and more calories even at rest. Don't just take my word for it. Research has proven this. Check this out:

✦ A recent study had college-age women perform resistance exercise for six weeks. The participants cut their body fat by as much as 13.7 percent, losing up to seven pounds of fat. They completely changed their bodies by lifting weights!

✦ In another study, 31 healthy women did periodized resistance training 5 days a week for 24 weeks. At the end of the six months, their body mass went down 2.2 percent, their body fat dropped by 10 percent, and their lean muscle tissue increased 2.2 percent. They got smaller and leaner, while boosting their metabolisms.

FIT FEMALE *Real Life Story*

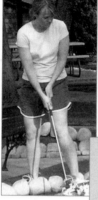

▲
Hillary 4 months after her son was born—her cardio queen body!

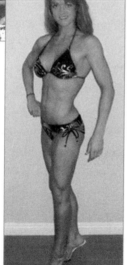

Hillary lost 25 pounds of fat and 4 sizes. ▶

Throughout my life, I had never really achieved the body I desired, which was developed and shapely. I got the running bug in my late teens or early twenties. I ran numerous 5-Ks and 10-Ks. I also trained for a couple of half marathons and a full marathon. I knew that lifting weights was important, but it came second to running. Any weight training was thrown in whenever I had time, and it was usually with pretty light weights.

While I trained for my first full marathon, I watched my body slowly become softer and even a little heavier. I never lost any weight, even with running those endless miles. I ate reasonably well and fueled my body for those long runs.

I continued running through my twenties and struggled with matching the body I had in my mind with what I was actually seeing in the mirror. I ran six to 10 miles five or six mornings a week.

At that time, I decided it was time to do something different: It was time to commit to lifting weights in addition to my running. I knew I needed to. I developed a program and stuck with it a few days a week. I was religious about running and lifting. The problem was I ran off all my hard work in the weight room. I wasn't about to drop the running, though. I was hoping my body would just start responding.

✦ Another study compared excess postexercise oxygen consumption (EPOC), which is what I refer to as the afterburn effect, after a treadmill workout and after a circuit workout of resistance-training exercises. The resistance-training circuit regimen prompted a significant increase in the number of calories the participants burned afterward, compared with the treadmill workout.

✦ Another study took place over 12 months using a program that included strength training and showed improved body composition, a decrease in waist circumference, and an increase in lean muscle. Weight

---

Then came pregnancy. Motherhood—I never would have thought it would bring the fit time of my life. Once I made it through the first trimester of my pregnancy, my doctor gave me the go-ahead to run. Running became jogging, and I continued to jog through my pregnancy without any problems. I gained the typical 25 to 30 pounds and felt pretty good.

After giving birth to our son, a week later I was at it again. I ran whenever I could, and when my son was big enough for a jogging stroller, he went along with me. About the time my son was four months old, something clicked in my brain.

I finally realized that I shouldn't run so much and instead needed to commit to lifting weights. Heavy weights.

We put together a home gym in our garage. It wasn't pretty, but it had the basics—squat rack, dumbbells, stability ball, chinup bar, and some bands. I quickly started to enjoy the feeling I had when I was finished working out. I stopped running altogether and started lifting. I got my workouts in very early before the baby woke, or during his nap time. It became a priority to me. I was a better mom and wife when I got my workout done.

After a month of training, I started to like what I was seeing in the mirror. I actually had shape to my muscles. I kept at it and began loving the results! My 30th birthday loomed in the future, and my goal was to look better in my thirties than I did in my twenties. In my workouts with Rachel, she not only reiterated the importance of letting my body build muscle by not doing so much cardio but also reinforced how important my diet was. I always ate fairly well, but she taught me that if I had my diet dialed in with my training, even better results would follow. With her expertise and a lot of hard work, I achieved my goal. I definitely look better in my thirties than I ever have in my life! I feel strong and love the body I've created. I have finally matched the image in my mind to the one I see in the mirror. I will continue to lift weights and make changes to my physique. I've learned that this chick belongs in the weight room. ✦

stayed the same. The participants did not get bulkier but instead got leaner and smaller and reinvented their bodies.

✦ One last study compared aerobic training with strength training. The aerobic group performed four hours of aerobics per week. The resistance group did 2 to 4 sets of 8 to 15 repetitions of 10 exercises, three times a week. Both groups lost weight. But the resistance-training group lost significantly more fat and didn't sacrifice any lean body mass, even eating only 800 calories a day. (The reason the calories were so low was to take any dietary variables completely out of the equation and compare the effects of the exercise regimes on lean body mass and metabolism.) The resistance-training group actually increased metabolism compared with the aerobic group, who decreased metabolism.

Using the right strength-training routine will give your body a metabolism boost that will create what I call a sizzling metabolism and an afterburn effect. Combining this with the right kind and amount of cardiovascular activity will turn your body into a fat-burning machine. Too much cardio works against you, because your body will eventually begin to utilize your hard-earned lean muscle tissue for energy, which is *not* the desired goal. If you watch any of the women who attend aerobics classes regularly over a six-month period, their bodies won't change at all for precisely this reason.

You have to stop pounding your body with aerobics and hours and hours of steady-state cardio, because you will lose muscle and slow your metabolism! Stop torturing yourself with exercise that feels like punishment, doing the same repetitive motions over and over again. Get out of the aerobics rooms, get off the treadmills and StairMasters, and start lifting weights. This fit female lifts weights, builds strength and definition, and keeps her metabolism high.

I know, I know . . . you've been misinformed and need help. You may not know what to do when it comes to lifting weights or how to lift weights properly. You feel silly when you venture onto the weight-training floor, because you don't know where to start. You can't tell if you're doing it right or if all the men are laughing at you because you don't know what you're doing. It can be intimidating, but that's why I'm here and this book is here—to help you gain the confidence you need to conquer the weight-training floor and become a fit female.

Even personal trainers can have it all wrong when it comes to training females. The majority of personal trainers are men, and when they get a female client, they think, "Ah, man, another 'toning' program." They give her light weights and lots of repetitions so she doesn't get too bulky. They try to give her shaping exercises so that she'll "feel the burn" in all the right spots. Really, that burn is just lactic acid building up because she's doing so many reps, but it doesn't mean anything. There is no toning or shaping, because nothing was done to actually challenge the muscles and make them build. These trainers' female clients never actually change their bodies, because they never gain any muscle. Even trainers are afraid to challenge women and push them to their limits. They don't realize women are capable of working hard and challenging themselves. Women actually have a higher pain tolerance than men. How is a female supposed to learn to lift weights right when even the "experts" tell her to use the light dumbbells for lots of reps or, worse, stick to aerobics? When most personal trainers they hire won't push them to challenge themselves enough in the gym?

I had a client who had been training with us for years and had completely changed her body and reinvented herself into a fit female. She loved to lift weights and had redefined her body with strength training. She had lost 40 pounds and was convinced of the benefits of lifting weights. She was so sad when her husband's job took them to the East Coast, because she didn't know what she was going to do without her gym. I reassured her that she would find another gym there and another trainer, and she would keep it up. A few weeks after she moved, she called me, really upset because she had been working with a trainer for a few weeks but he refused to give her challenging weights because she would "bulk up," in his words. He had her doing lots of cardio and no weight training. She was losing her fit female body and was frustrated that he wasn't giving her a strength program and letting her lift weights. Of course, I thought it was ridiculous that she was telling this trainer that she wanted to lift heavier because she knew it would make her body look better and that he ignored her. She was trying to convince him that strength training was how she lost 40 pounds of fat and that she needed to lift. And he, the fitness professional, was talking her out of it . . . talking her out of pushing herself in the gym and challenging her body.

This was a big wake-up call to me as far as what we women are up against when it comes to learning how to lift weights properly and reap the benefits of strength training.

Maybe there's a conspiracy among all the men to tell women strength training will make us big and bulky to keep us off the weights, because it's their secret mission to make the weight room less crowded. Well, we are on to you, men . . . aren't we, girls?

Everyone knows men have an easier time losing weight than women do. If you've ever had a weight-loss contest with your significant other, you know he always has an advantage. Why is this the case? Could it be that he has more lean body mass and therefore a higher metabolic rate? As a woman, you'll never get your lean body mass as high as his because of your biological makeup, but you can increase your lean body mass to even out the game some and get the benefits of an increased metabolism.

One thing to think about when it comes to women and exercise is that we have been conditioned to look at exercise through the prism of what we can't do. Think about it. Men, for their entire lives, work out with the mindset that they can do anything and can always do more, meaning get stronger, bigger, faster, leaner, and so on. They are never told that they can't. Women, however, have always been told that we can't—we can't do real pushups, so we should do "girl pushups"; we can't do chinups; we can't lift heavy weights. The list goes on. It all starts when girls are young and are told to do "girl pushups" instead of real pushups "because you're a girl." And so most women don't do anything other than a "girl pushup" for the rest of their lives, thinking, *I'm a girl—I can't do a real pushup!* In fact, the first woman to run a marathon had to disguise herself as a man because women "can't do marathons."

Go to any women-only section of a gym and you'll see rinky-dink dumbbells, probably up to 15 pounds (less than the weight of most handbags), and of course those stupid inner-thigh machines that must have been created by a man to do nothing but give the guys a nice crotch shot! There is nothing there to challenge a woman to work out and change her body.

Lifting weights give you the body you've always wanted, but there are so many other reasons you should incorporate strength training into your life. In fact, there are many more benefits for women who lift weights than there are for men. What I don't understand is why more women aren't lifting weights. If having the body you want doesn't motivate you to push yourself in the gym with challenging weights, then the following information should.

Besides changing the way their bodies look, other benefits women are missing out on when they don't lift weights include:

+ **Completely stopping and reversing bone loss.** You can actually reverse bone loss using strength training. This may not be a worry for you right now, but starting to lift weights now will set you up to have strong bones down the road. Bone mass usually decreases as we age. Lifting weights can actually help you increase it. This is also something to keep in mind when you're focused on that number on the scale—your bone weighs something, and as you are getting stronger, so are your bones, which will add weight to the scale. Just remember that this is a good thing! There have been numerous studies showing that weight-bearing exercise increases bone mass. One in particular

OLD-SCHOOL STRENGTH

Did you know that the legendary Marilyn Monroe lifted weights? She was a girl before her time but knew that being strong and lifting weights would give her the body she wanted.

was a one-year study that used a strength-training routine three days a week and showed that in women, the more weight they lifted, the greater the increase in total-body bone density. Another study done in 2007 had young women participate for five months in a resistance-training program, and the conclusion was that strength training increased bone mass. A third study, done in 2000, showed that the positive effects of resistance training on the musculoskeletal system reverse when training is withdrawn. If you don't use it, you lose it! Real life story: One of my clients actually had a bone density scan done right before she started lifting weights and found out that she was at medium risk of bone loss. She started lifting weights, and after a year she had the scan done again, which showed amazing results: She had gone from medium to low risk for bone loss. Her bone density had increased by 13 percent—that's more than 1 percent a month on average! And she lost 65 pounds of fat over that year! She gained bone and lost fat by lifting weights!

✦ **Decreasing your risk of injuries.** You can't be a fit female if you're injured. Having a stronger, fitter body will decrease your risk of injury in sports and in everyday activities. Women have a higher incidence of anterior cruciate ligament (ACL) tears than men do, but using a strength-training program can decrease the risk of this. Women tend to have hypermobile joints and need more stability to prevent injuries. The only way to create more stability is to add strength. Numerous studies have shown that women are four to six times more likely than men to sustain a knee injury, such as an ACL tear. A study done in 2007 confirmed previous studies showing that female athletes substantially decrease their risk of an ACL injury when they use resistance training.

✦ **Boosting your stamina and function in everyday activities.** You may have a rigorous schedule that includes picking up kids, grocery shopping, doing the laundry, and cooking dinner, along with holding down a job and/or going to school. A study published in 2007 showed that women who did a heavy resistance-training program improved their economy of physical activity, including functioning in daily tasks, which increased their quality of life. This study also showed that their body mass didn't increase: Participants' weight stayed the same, but they all lost body fat. Once again, weight training helps you function better, but it doesn't make you bigger. Using the programs in this book, you will notice a definite difference in how you feel every day as you take care of all your responsibilities.

✦ **Reversing the aging process.** Yes! You *can* turn back the clock! The average woman starts losing 8 to 10 percent of her strength each decade starting around age 40, according to Len Kravitz, Ph.D. We can reverse this with strength training! Fast-twitch fibers contract quickly and are well adapted to perform anaerobic exercise such as strength training, whereas slow-twitch muscle fibers contract more slowly. As you age these fast-twitch fibers are the first to go and are what are most important in keeping you moving like a young person. Research has shown that you can increase muscle firing rates after just one week of training. With more muscles firing especially fast-twitch ones, you have more energy for life. According to a review done in 2009 and published in the *Journal of Applied Physiology,* resistance training not only delays muscle loss for decades, but can actually reverse it and is effective at increasing skeletal muscle mass and improving functional performance in the elderly. Women who work their muscles retain significantly more strength as they get older. Be young and fabulous!

◆ **Increasing self-esteem and feeling empowered.** This is by far the most important benefit of lifting weights. Strength training increases self-esteem and confidence, and will positively affect everything else in your life, including your relationships, your career, and whatever else you allow it to flow into. Even your sex drive will be higher!

Most women don't realize they can reduce their risk of injuries and osteoporosis and speed up their metabolisms while losing fat, feeling younger, functioning better in daily life, boosting their self-esteem, and feeling good about themselves, all by making strength training part of their routine. All it takes is a (confident) stride to the strength-training floor. What are you waiting for?

WHAT IS METABOLISM?

Throughout this book, I talk about boosting your metabolism and getting your body burning more fat to produce what I call a sizzling metabolism. One of my clients started following my principles and said to me, "I'm hungry all the time!" I said, "That's your metabolism picking up. That is a good sign that you're burning a lot of calories and therefore fat." She said, "What exactly is this thing called metabolism you speak of? Where is it? How does it work? Why do we want it to be high?"

Metabolism, as defined in the dictionary, is the sum of the physical and chemical processes in the body by which its material substance is produced, maintained, and destroyed, and by which energy is made available. Huh? Basically, metabolism is everything going on in your body added up. Metabolism is how many calories a day your body burns to do what it does every day. Your metabolism without doing any activity, just lying on the couch all day, is called your basal metabolic rate and can be anywhere from 1,200 calories a day on up. We want to get yours *up!* The goal, in order to turn you into a fit female, is to stoke your metabolism as high as possible. As we boost your metabolism, you will become a fat-burning machine with a sizzling metabolism.

Sizzling metabolism: A metabolism that burns (sizzles) a large amount of energy (fat) every day to function in life.

What will boost your metabolism to make it sizzle? Doing an intense workout, having more muscle tissue, and eating frequently are easy ways to boost your metabolism. Later on, I'll give you tools and strategies to ratchet up your metabolism and get it revving to where you're hungry all the time, because your body is burning through everything, including your body fat. Remember, that's a *good* thing! The goal of this program is to get you to the point where your body burns a ton of calories every day, you fuel your body with healthy food all day long, you have energy, and you're fit and fabulous, with a sizzling metabolism that won't stop.

BUT CAN'T I JUST GO RUNNING?

I know what you're thinking: All this lifting and metabolic stuff . . . can't I just go out for a run and get fit? I used to think the same thing. The first person to teach me about aerobics not being effective for fat loss was my husband, Alwyn Cosgrove. I remember when I first met

him and he said this to me, and I kept asking him, "But what if I *want* to go for a run?" He would say, "What is your goal?" I would say, "To lose fat." He would say, "Then don't go for a run." "But what if I just want to go running?" . . . We went in circles until I realized what he was saying to me—don't run to lose fat. You can run because you like to run, but don't run to accomplish your goal of losing fat. It won't help. It all clicked, and I realized the years and years I had been teaching aerobics classes and going for runs were all making my body hold on to fat rather than burn it. This was why I had never achieved my fit female body . . . until I started lifting weights and pushing myself with intervals.

Now, years later, in my experience, I've realized that the average woman starting a fitness program has no business running. That's right, no business! Running is actually an extremely advanced exercise. January 1, you see hundreds of New Year's resolutioners hitting the streets to start their new year right by going for a run!

When did running become the starting point for someone who wants to get in shape? It drives me crazy when I hear someone say, "I want to come to your gym, but first I'm going to start running to lose some weight on my own." I just want to shake them and say, "Don't you realize running is very hard and very advanced? Running is actually extremely ineffective as a weight-loss modality. You'll end up coming to me three months from now

DEBUNKING THE MYTHS

Myth #1: Women will get big and bulky if they lift heavy weights. Using strength training will build some muscle, so if you're scared of looking firmer, toned, and fit, you shouldn't touch a weight. But no woman I have worked with has ever become big, huge, and bulky. Using the right program will give you definition and the right amount of muscle size as you're losing fat, so you'll be smaller, with toned arms and a hard butt and thighs. The only way to look fit is to build some muscle. You can't be afraid of muscle. Most men have a hard time getting big and bulky, and *they have 10 to 30 times more testosterone than we do*. A woman will not look like a man as a result of lifting weights.

You're probably asking, "What about those bodybuilder women who look like men? Isn't that from lifting heavy weights?" No! Any woman who looks like a man looks that way because she is using something else to enhance her hormonal makeup to be more like that of a man, increasing her testosterone to the point that she gains muscle as easily as a man does. So her body responds to weights more like a man's body would. If you are not taking steroids and chemically enhancing yourself in order to have the hormonal makeup of a man, your body will never look like that of a man. They actually figured this out way back in 1974 (where have we been, girls?), when a study was done to evaluate changes in strength, body composition, and muscular hypertrophy resulting from a six-month strength-training program using near-maximal resistance exercises in women. The women did three days a week of strength training and kept their diets the same. All the women showed substantial increases in their strength and were able to lift more at the end than when they started, but despite this, they actually lost fat and did not gain any size during the study. In a more recent study done in 2001, researchers had young women whose average age was 22 perform total-body strength-training workouts three days a week for six months. There was absolutely no change in body mass (the participants did not get any bigger), but their body fat on aver-

age went from 26.5 percent to 19.8 percent, and their lean body mass increased on average by seven pounds over the six months. They did not get bigger but completely changed their body composition. Get ready to push yourself in the gym. Lift enough weight to build muscle and watch your body change into that of a fit female.

Myth #2: Women should be careful about lifting too heavy. You've heard it before—"Let me get that for you; you're a girl." Oh, that makes me mad—I can get it! Or "You should be careful; it's dangerous for a woman to lift that much weight." Are we fragile, weak individuals? No! It's important to have a strong body, and if you progress properly with the right program, you won't get hurt. Most of my clients lift 30- to 40-pound kids several times a day. How are we going to get this same woman's body to change by handing her a pink Barbie dumbbell that weighs 3 pounds? She needs to lift weights, and more than she's already used to. Heck, most handbags weigh close to 20 pounds.

Myth #3: Women get all the benefits they need from running or other aerobic activities. Seriously, let's think about what the average woman does in a day—picks up kids a couple of times, lifts 20-pound grocery bags, loads laundry with a twisting action, and then carries it as an offset load up the stairs. . . . How the heck does running in one plane of motion get any woman ready for the activities she does on a day-to-day basis, let alone cause her body to change? Research has shown that total-body resistance training enhances the total fitness profile by increasing strength in upper-body muscles and improving muscle performance, and by boosting cardiovascular fitness more than aerobics alone can.

Myth #4: Women should do the same programs as men do. Why do women try to train exactly the same way as men? It fails. Women don't need to isolate their biceps or blitz their pecs. Women have different goals. They need a program designed specifically for women. That doesn't necessarily mean an easy program—and don't worry, no pink dumbbells are involved.

weighing the same, but with an injury from your running."

I have been an endurance athlete, and I have coached endurance athletes, so why would I be so against running for the average woman? Besides coaching endurance athletes, I've also coached more than a thousand women in the gym whose No. 1 goal is to lose fat and get in shape. Many of these women are average women who are not active and are not runners but want to look fit. With this type of clientele, average women, I would never, ever start them off on day one, workout one, with 1,500 reps of a one-legged plyometric (jumping) exercise. In all my education in exercise prescriptions, I was always taught that plyometrics are an advanced exercise that shouldn't be used until a client at least had a base strength built up. Forget 1,500 reps. Running for one mile is exactly this—1,500 reps (steps) of a plyometric exercise. Running produces forces in the area of two to five times your body weight per foot contact. So now we're talking 1,500 reps with two to five times your body weight on each rep. Pretty advanced stuff for day one, workout one, don't you think?

Sixty-five percent of all runners have to stop running and seek treatment due to overuse injuries. Of this 65%, female runners have been shown to be more susceptible, especially to stress fractures, than male runners. I believe that running can be damaging and very hard on the body, especially for a beginning exerciser. But if someone has been working out consistently, building strength in the weight room, and is fit enough to run and handle two to three times their body weight for 1,500 reps, *then* they can add a couple of running workouts per week to their fitness program. First they have to get fit enough to do this and earn the right to take up an advanced exercise such as running. It's just like wearing a belly-baring top—you have to earn the right to wear a belly-baring top. Certain people have not put in the training and dieting to be allowed to wear a belly-baring top. Hint: If you have a muffin top (you know, that roll that hangs over your pants), you are not allowed to wear a belly-baring top. Similarly, if you're not fit enough and have not been following a strength-training program, you are not allowed to run. No belly-baring tops and no running! Get in the gym first and earn both! And once you've put in some strength training and have earned it, unless you have a goal of completing an endurance event, these sessions should not be longer than three to four miles at a time.

"You can't run to get fit, you need to be fit to run."
—DIANE LEE

That brings me to my next point. What is your goal? If your goal is to complete an endurance event in which you have to run, then by all means run. Your training needs to include running, and you'd better make sure you've done some strength training. You'll have to put in time foam-rolling and stretching. Above all, you have to be sure you're fit enough to start running. Completing a 5-K, a half marathon, or even a marathon is an excellent goal, but you need to make sure you're fit enough to run first.

Or is your goal weight loss or to look like a fit female? Running is not necessary in order to look like a fit female. Most people who run have a goal of losing weight or getting that "runner's body." I hate to be the one to break it to you, but running will not give you a runner's body. In fact, if you're not fit enough to run, you'll end up injured, and you'll have to sit on the couch with your injury and get farther away from your runner's body. Quoting a strength coach who has worked with many successful female athletes, Mike Boyle, "Women who run successfully for long periods of time were made to run. They look just like men runners. Good female runners generally do not look like plus-size models. It's not a question of cause and effect; it's a question of natural selection. You can't run to get that cute little runner's body. It's actually reversed. You have to have that cute little runner's body to survive running."

BUT WHY DO THEY CALL IT THE "FAT-BURNING ZONE"?

During a steady-state aerobic workout (in which you move at the same pace for a certain amount of time), your body does burn a higher *percentage* of calories from fat. This is where that "fat-burning zone" myth comes from. On the surface, it sounds as if you're burning more calories of fat overall.

There are two big problems with this.

1. The first problem is that your body will adapt quickly. And as your body adapts, you burn fewer *total* calories. So even if you're burning a higher *percentage* of fat, you aren't burning as many calories overall, because it's a higher percentage of a smaller number. It's like winning 80 percent of a Lotto jackpot. You're all excited until you realize that the jackpot is only 50 bucks.

2. The other problem is that your body actually becomes an efficient fat-*storing* machine. Since you're now burning fat as your primary source of fuel, your body adapts and becomes very good at storing fat. (Unfortunately, our bodies are very smart.) If your car is fuel efficient, it burns less gas. Same with your body: As it becomes more efficient, you burn less fuel (fat is stored fuel) to do the same work. Not ideal.

I do not use any form of steady-state, "fat-burning zone" training with my fat-loss clients. I've found that using a full-body resistance-training program with shorter rest periods along with two or three metabolic interval-training sessions a week is the most effective for fat loss. The goal for fat loss is to get your metabolism up. Your body adapts extremely quickly to steady-state cardio, and you'll burn fewer and fewer calories the more of it you do. With interval training, your metabolism will be up for the next 24 to 48 hours, giving you an afterburn effect. Going for a run will not necessarily get you closer to your goal of looking fit. Just check out the finish line of any endurance event. You'll see bodies of all shapes and sizes.

So, are you still determined to run? Or have I done a good job of talking you out of it? I don't necessarily want to talk you out of running, but I want to make you aware that it is an advanced exercise. It's not for out-of-shape beginners trying to get in shape. There are better choices. My point is this: If you are a woman who simply wants to look leaner, lose fat, and be a fit female, running does not have to be a part of your routine. On the other hand, if you have a goal of completing an endurance event or you simply enjoy running, be aware that it is an advanced exercise, and be sure to get fit enough to run.

THE FINAL NAIL IN THE AEROBICS COFFIN

In my case, the final nail in the coffin of steady-state aerobics for fat loss was when I trained for and completed an Ironman Triathlon. When I started training for it, I thought surely with all the training I was about to do, even though it would be steady state, I would get into even better shape than I was in already.

I had been lifting weights and had done some shorter triathlons and was able to maintain my fit female body. But by the time I was ready to complete my Ironman, my body was soft, with no definition, and had *definitely* changed due to spending the majority of my training in the steady-state aerobic zone—the same "fat-burning zone" many books and magazines still talk about.

I was in great shape as far as my endurance and cardiovascular system were concerned, but I had less noticeable muscle tone and no longer had the definition I was used to having in my abs and arms.

Put it this way: I didn't even want to wear a crop top at my race, because I didn't have abs to show. I'd lost some muscle and looked soft and flabby, but I was still happy with my performance and thrilled that I accomplished my goal.

All my training was done in order to prepare to complete an Ironman, and the purpose of eating was to fuel me for the workouts. At the time, my goal wasn't to lose fat, but I was still amazed at how *little* fat I lost.

I worked my way up to doing 20 hours of endurance training a week. I also kept track of every calorie I ate, making sure my nutrition was right on track. I thought I'd be able to eat whatever I wanted, but I couldn't. I had to watch myself to keep from gaining any weight.

Some of the workouts included eight- or nine-hour sessions in which I'd go for a 10-mile run, then jump on my bike for a 70-mile ride and finish with a four-mile run. I also continued to lift weights twice a week, in an effort to maintain *some* muscle tone but also to stay injury free and somewhat strong.

My body quickly adapted, and I was able to increase my mileage until I could go for a 16-mile run or a 112-mile bike ride as if it were "just another workout." It was amazing to see how the body adapts to demands and how far you can push yourself.

Unfortunately, this was also exactly why I didn't lose much fat—my body *was* adapting to what I was doing. My goal was to make my body superefficient at running 20 miles and riding a bike 100 miles, so when it came time for my race, I'd be able to do it.

However, the more your body adapts, the fewer calories you burn. So I was doing more and more exercise without burning as many calories, and therefore I wasn't losing any fat.

In seven months of training, I calculated that I worked out for 374 hours—that's an average of more than 12 hours a week! If I burned just 10 calories a minute, it adds up to 224,400 calories. Doing the math (at 3,500 calories per pound), 224,400 calories *should* equal 64 pounds lost! Needless to say, I did *not* lose 64 pounds. Over those seven months, training an average of 12 to 14 hours a week, I lost all of *five* pounds. That. Was. It.

Fortunately, I now have firsthand experi-ence confirming that steady-state aerobics is absolutely, completely, utterly ineffective for fat loss. After working my way up to 20 training hours a week, I can tell you that long, steady-state endurance is *not* the answer for a defined, lean physique, and it's a waste of time if your goal is fat loss. It's the answer *only* if your goal is to complete an endurance event.

LEARN TO LOVE INTENSITY, NOT DURATION

There is actually a ton of research that shows that steady-state aerobics doesn't work for fat loss, and interval training does. Let's review some of it.

✦ The landmark study on interval training pitted 20 weeks of endurance training against 15 weeks of interval training. The energy cost of the endurance training equaled 28,661 calories, while the energy cost of the interval training came to 13,614 calories (less than half). Yet the interval-training group showed a *nine times greater* loss of subcutaneous fat than the endurance group (when corrected for energy cost).

✦ In 1998, a study had women do 45 minutes of aerobic exercise at 78 percent of maximum heart rate five days a week for 12 weeks. It showed *no effect* on body composition beyond what was accomplished with dieting alone.

✦ In 2007, a six-month study was published showing that adding aerobic exercise for 50 minutes five days a week had no additional effect on body composition, beyond diet alone.

✦ In December 2006, Canadian researchers reported that seven sessions of high-intensity interval training over two weeks increased women's fat-burning enzymes, boosting their ability to burn fat during exercise by 36 percent.

✦ In June 2007, a 12-month study was published that had the subjects doing six hours of aerobic exercise per week, training six days a week, for one year. The average weight loss was only three pounds during that one-year period—that is, only a quarter of a pound per month. Losing three pounds over a one-year period is pretty insignificant. This was a lot of exercise for very little result, especially when you look at the results of the next study.

✦ In a study done in 2008, Australian researchers had 18 women perform 20 minutes of interval training on a stationary bike three days a week: eight seconds of sprinting followed by 12 seconds of recovery. The women lost an average of 5½ pounds over 15 weeks, without dieting. Similar groups performing 40 minutes of steady-state cycling three days a week actually *gained* a pound of fat over the same period. Two of the heavier women

who did intervals dropped 18 pounds. Now, those are the results I'm talking about!

✦ According to a British study done in 2002, levels of human growth hormone, which assists in increasing lean muscle and burning fat, skyrocketed 530 percent in subjects after just 30 seconds of sprinting as fast as they could on a stationary bike.

✦ Yet another study had overweight subjects assigned to three groups: diet only, diet plus aerobics, and diet plus aerobics plus weights. The diet-only group lost 14.6 pounds of fat in 12 weeks. The aerobics group (who did 30 minutes three times a week and progressed to 50 minutes) lost only one more pound (15.6 pounds) than the diet group. The weight-training group lost 21.1 pounds of fat! That's 35 percent more than the diet and aerobics group! Basically, the addition of aerobic exercise didn't result in any significant results over dieting alone. Thirty-six sessions of up to 50 minutes is a lot of work for one additional pound of fat loss. However, the addition of resistance training greatly accelerated fat-loss results.

UNDOING THE AEROBIC DAMAGE

After completing my Ironman, I switched gears and made fat loss my primary goal for eight weeks. I eliminated *all* steady-state endurance exercise. No running, biking, swimming, or anything else in the steady state.

My workouts consisted of high intensity for short bursts, whether it was lifting weights or doing a metabolic interval session. I lifted weights three days a week and performed interval-training workouts on the other days.

I made sure the interval workouts weren't on a treadmill or a bike, since my body was so adapted to these. I used only body-weight metabolic circuits (like the ones in this book) as my cardio workouts.

These metabolic cardio workouts would crank up my heart rate for two minutes, I'd recover, and then repeat. Doing these interval circuits, along with strength training, took up a total of five to six hours a week—nothing like the 20 to 30 hours of Ironman training! What happened? Like magic, my abs came back!

I dropped 15 pounds of fat in an eight-week period, and my body returned to being strong, defined, and lean. I no longer looked flabby, and I did it in a quarter of the time, compared with the aerobic training.

IT WORKS, BUT WHY?

One reason intervals are more effective is that they target more of your muscle. During endurance exercise, you use a lot of slow-twitch muscle fibers and too *few* fast-twitch muscle fibers. It's those fast-twitch muscle fibers that give you firm muscles and fast-tracked results.

Now, don't get me wrong, I still enjoy heading out for a run or a bike ride occasionally, but I don't do it for fat loss. I do it because I enjoy it. Think about it. If you do a 30-minute walk at a steady-state, moderate pace, you'll burn about 150 calories.

If you mix in eight 30-second sprints, you'll burn closer to 200 calories. But the biggest factor is that after an interval session, your metabolism can stay elevated for a full day, and you'll end up burning two to three times the total calories you'd expect to burn through lower-intensity exercise. That is the goal of the training plan in this book.

A study in the *European Journal of Applied Physiology* proved this, using a circuit-training program of 12 sets in 31 minutes. EPOC was elevated significantly for 38 hours postworkout. Thirty-eight hours is a pretty significant time frame for metabolism to be elevated. If you trained from 9:00 to 10:00 on Monday morning, you'd still be burning more calories (without additional training) at midnight on Tuesday!

It's time to bury, for good, the myth that long, slow, steady-state cardio will burn fat. No more spending hours and hours on the treadmill, elliptical trainer, or bike.

R.I.P., AEROBICS

Get off the treadmill, stop spinning your wheels, and *push* yourself in the gym if you want to lose some serious fat. Take it from me—I finally learned firsthand. It's time to put the last nail in the coffin of using aerobics for fat loss, bury it for good, and do some high-intensity interval dancing on its overdue grave.

Part 2

REINVENTING YOURSELF

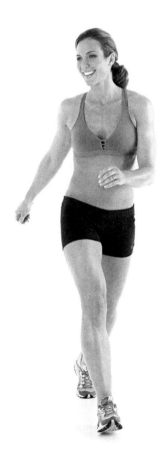

Chapter 4

Deciding What You Want and Why

THE FIT FEMALE WITHIN

It's time to get serious and get focused. If I'm right about you, you didn't buy this book to skim through it, put it on your bookshelf, and let another year go by during which you don't achieve the absolute ultimate body you have always dreamed of having. Within this book is everything you need to finally make the breakthrough and become the confident, empowered, fit female you've always thought about becoming but have had trouble making a reality. How can you be sure you'll take action this time and stay motivated to finally reach the body you want? Take on this challenge with a different attitude. To achieve success, you must change your mindset and decide this will be it and you will become a fit female. Decide that you will do what it takes!

"Goal setting can be so powerful. It provides focus. It shapes our dreams. It gives us the ability to hone in on the exact actions we need to do to get everything that we desire in life."

　　　　　　　　　　　　　　　　—JIM ROHN

You can start by looking in the mirror and asking yourself some tough questions. Be honest with yourself and really think about the following questions. Don't just read them. Answer them.

You picked up this book because you're looking for something. Is it a feeling you're after? Is it a look you want? Whatever it is, it is within you. Start to peel back the layers to get to who you really want to become. Do you want to fit into your skinny jeans again? Do you want to feel sexy and be able to wear whatever you want with confidence? Do you want more energy? Or maybe you're tired of feeling ashamed of the way you look, and you want to feel fit and empowered in your own body. Do you want to feel better in clothes? Or maybe out of clothes? Why did you pick up this book? Write your answers here.

_____

_____

Bottom line: Are you ready to change and become the person you want to be? Are you ready to do what it takes?

_____

_____

Why now?

_____

_____

What has kept you from following through and making these changes in the past?

_____

_____

Are those obstacles still a problem?

_____

_____

What motivates you?

_____

_____

"If you don't go after what you want, you'll never have it. If you don't ask, the answer is always no. If you don't step forward, you're always in the same place."

—NORA ROBERTS

If you really want to change your body and become a fit female who feels empowered, confident, and sexy, you have to decide that you want it and why you want it. Know what drives you and what will keep you motivated. The questions you just answered should help you to reflect and get you thinking about who you are and what it would mean to you to change your body. This is a simple process yet absolutely critical to achieving the body of your dreams. Once you successfully complete the exercises in this chapter, you'll be ready to embark on your quest of becoming a fit female. The rest will come easily, and you'll enjoy the process of transforming your body, empowering your mind, and feeling sexy and confident. If you ignore this step, you are destined to fail, no matter how good the nutrition and training advice in this book is. Most people won't take the time and instead will open this book and go straight to the training program, grocery list, and menus, looking for the "answer" or the magic trick. These same people will get only a few weeks into the program before they lose motivation, and they will be destined to fail because they never took the time to examine why they wanted to change in the first place and, more important, what they were willing to do to achieve that change.

Having a clearly defined goal gives you a destination to aim for, but this isn't enough on its own. You also need to have a powerful driving force—an understanding of *why* you want to accomplish that goal—which will create a magnet that will pull you toward that destination. You will undoubtedly encounter obstacles over the course of your journey—everybody does. However, if you don't know exactly where it is you're going and why you want to go there, you'll easily be pulled off track, and the smallest obstacle will cause you to give up. (Reread Secret #8 in the Fit Female Credo.) But if you know exactly where you're going, what you want to look like, how you want to feel, and what clothes you want to wear—and you have a powerful reason why—you can get through any obstacle, because the magnet will be strong enough to pull you toward your goal, making it easier not to give up until you get there.

So, let's make some decisions. Use a pencil.

Without considering whether it's realistic, write down what you absolutely want to achieve during this journey. No limits! Be very specific. Define what becoming a fit female means to you. How will you know you've reached your goal? (Example: I will wear a size 8 and throw away all my "fat" clothes, and never feel insecure about my body again.)

_____

_____

What are you willing to do to make this a reality for you? What sacrifices are you willing to make? Are you willing to give up your favorite food? Are you ready to get up earlier in the morning? Will you make time to plan your day ahead? Skip your nightly ice cream? Are you ready to do what you need to do to reach the above goal?

_____

_____

If the above goal is not important enough to you to make sacrifices, than you need to rethink it. Make sure your goal is one that you *must* accomplish, not just one that you *should* accomplish. Erase and rewrite your goal if the latter is the case. (That's why you used pencil.)

_____

_____

What sacrifices are you absolutely *not* willing to make? What will you not give up? Will this keep you from reaching the above goal?

_____

_____

How will you feel the day you are a fit female, wearing the clothes you want to wear, feeling the way you want to feel, with boundless energy, living a fulfilling life and ready to take on anything? What will this mean to you?

_____

_____

The most important thing is that you really understand what your driving force is and why the goal is important. Why is it a "must" instead of a "should"? What will drive you to do what it takes? What will be the repercussions if you do not become the fit female you want to become?

_____

_____

Thinking about everything you've answered above, come up with your fit female mission statement. This should be a phrase that is easy to remember and sums up your motivation and reason why. This phrase will be your mantra throughout your transformation.

Examples: "There is no time like the present."
"No more excuses."
"Nothing to it but to do it."
"I am fit and fabulous."
"Keep moving forward."
"I am strong beyond belief; I am powerful beyond measure."
"A strong outside strengthens the inside."

_____

_____

_____

Time to visualize. This is a very important step in this process. Do not skip it! I don't care how silly you think it is. You have to tap into the way you will look and feel, and visualize it. Close your eyes right now and picture yourself as a fit female. When you first do this, it may be very tough to do, and you may not be able to see a clear picture of what you'll look and feel like. It may be fuzzy, or you may not be able to picture it at all. Keep practicing. Every day, close your eyes and picture it. Get a clear picture in your head of how you want to look and feel. This will take practice. I have had clients tell me the picture looks as if they're under water, as if they can kind of see it, but not really. With practice, it becomes more and more clear.

Fit Female Visual Tool

Once you have a clear picture of what you'll feel like, what you'll look like, what you'll wear, and how empowered and confident you'll be, make a fist with your right hand while you have the picture in your head. Start to connect that vision with your fist. This is a very powerful tool for when you may be tempted to make an excuse. Anytime you need to refocus, simply close your eyes and make a fist, and the vision will pop into your head, reminding you of the feeling you'll have when you reach your goal. One of my clients told me she was at a buffet party and everyone was eating and drinking. She'd been so focused on her goal and feeling so good, but she started to think about taking one night off and enjoying the food and drinks. However, she stopped herself, closed her eyes for a second, and made a fist, and her vision popped into her head. She had a great time at the party without eating or drinking anything she knew would sabotage her progress, and she came home feeling even more empowered because she had not given in. She came in the gym the next day exclaiming, "It worked! The fist worked!"

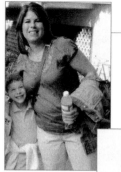

▲
Lisa before

**Lisa as a fit
female—lost
40 pounds
of fat and
4 clothing
sizes.** ▶

FIT FEMALE *Real Life Story*

"I feel empowered through exercise and getting in shape. I recently had someone come up to me and say, "You look great—you look like you've been working out!" Not just "You look like you've lost weight." That's what makes this experience different from anything else I've ever done. This program was never just about weight loss. This, for me, is about changing my body, empowering my body and my mind, and just feeling good again." ✦

Chapter 5

Overcoming a Self-Destructive Relationship with Food

FOOD IS A DRUG. DO YOU HAVE AN ADDICTION?

You can't reinvent yourself without first addressing your relationship with food. I can give you all the nutrition advice in the world and lay out exactly how you should eat, but if you don't get your head in the right place first, none of it will work. You have to acknowledge and start working on this relationship with food. For many of you, a lifetime of dieting, starving yourself, bingeing, beating yourself up, and losing and gaining weight has probably taken its toll. We need to work on this first.

Women and their relationship with food: Where do we start? Food is very emotional for women. Most women have a love-hate relationship with food. In this book, I hope to completely change your mindset and help you to build a healthy relationship with food. This is not going to be easy, because most of you have had this dysfunctional relationship with food for years. But if you're ready to change that relationship, this will be your breakthrough and a turning point for many of you.

"My mood will not affect my food."

—ONE OF MY CLIENTS, CINDY SCHEER

MY OWN RELATIONSHIP WITH FOOD

Thinking back to when I was 12 years old, I remember my dance instructor telling me that I was a very good dancer but that I didn't have a dancer's body, and that would hold me back. My dance instructor was someone I respected,

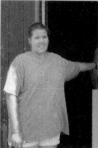

▲
Heather before

Heather as a fit female, after losing 60 pounds of fat and 6 clothing sizes. She is ecstatic that she no longer has to shop for plus sizes.

FIT FEMALE *Real Life Story*

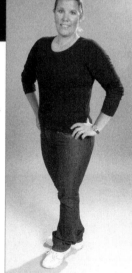

I have struggled with my weight all my life. I'm an emotional eater. I eat when I'm sad, stressed, or even happy. Food was my comfort. After two complicated pregnancies and having a child with special needs, I maxed out on my weight gain. I always put my family first. I did not know how to put myself first. Between stress and excess weight, I was suffering from high blood pressure. I realized that to take better care of my family, I had to put my health first. I had watched family members fight to win the battle against cancer, and here I was, unhealthy just from food.

I went to Rachel, and she had me write a commitment to myself. I had never put it in writing before. Doing that made it seem real to me. I started eating healthily and working out three days a week. My goal was to get healthy and lower my blood pressure. My doctors were blown away by how healthy I became in a short amount of time. I have now gone from being a couch potato to finishing a marathon, a half-marathon, and eight triathlons, and I have one healthy, fit body. ✦

so I took what she said very seriously. Of course, staring into a mirror comparing myself to the other girls in class didn't help, either. I wasn't fat; I was "athletic" and "big boned." I had a bigger frame than most of the other dancers. I was a mesomorph, so I had more muscle, and as my body developed, I had hips and curves. I did not have a typical, waiflike dancer's body, and I never would have one.

Combine this with the fact that I watched my mom struggle with her weight her entire life, going on and off diets, trying to find the answer to losing weight, only to gain it back every time. My brother and sister were also overweight. I knew I did not want to struggle for the rest of my life the way my mom strug-gles with her weight. I quickly started to read and learn about nutrition and working out. I started keeping a food journal, in which I would count my calories and grams of fat—meticulously tracking everything that went into my mouth, restricting myself, obsessing. Aa-a-ahh, this was the start of my adverse relationship with food. I would be in total control of everything, and then something would trigger me, and I would be totally out of control. This behavior turned into a binge eating disorder, where I would find myself "checking out," as I call it, or unconsciously eating and bingeing on the nearest trigger food I could get my hands on until I felt sick and horrible. And inevitably I ended up beating myself up. I remember thinking, "I'll just eat as much as I want of whatever I want right now, and I'll get back on my diet tomorrow, back in control—strict!" It was always a temporary thing in my head. I always thought that this would be the last time I would do this, and then I would be in control from then on.

Eventually, this turned into bulimia. I realized that I could get rid of that sick feeling and not worry about gaining any weight by making myself throw up. Off to the bathroom I would go to stick my finger down my throat. In my head, it would be as if it never happened. I wouldn't have to feel guilty about losing control of my diet. I struggled with bulimia at the end of high school, into college, and even after college. Temporary it was not. For at least five years, this happened on and off. Nobody knew

OFF-ON-A-TANGENT SIDE NOTE

Pilates will not give you a dancer's body. One of my pet peeves is the claim that Pilates will give you a dancer's body. Occasionally some-one will say to me, "I do Pilates to get long, lean dancer's muscles." People who have danc-er's bodies are born with dancer's bodies, and all the dancers who do Pilates looked like that when they walked in. Pilates started as rehab, and then they started marketing it to the aver-age consumer, stating that it will give you a dancer's body. No exercise will lengthen your muscles and give you longer legs. (Believe me, I would have done it by now.) Your muscles are the length they are, and you can't change that. Just as running won't give you a runner's body, dancing won't give you a dancer's body—nei-ther will Pilates.

The goal is to get your best body, which most likely is not a runner's or a dancer's body but your own fit female body!

I had this going on—my college roommates reading this are probably very surprised right now. I was very good at eating healthily in public and working out, and then I would binge by myself and throw it up. As I learned more in college about health and the long-term damage bulimia causes, I threw up less and less but would still binge occasionally. And, every once in a while, I'd find myself in the bathroom throwing up. Why was I doing this when I knew how unhealthy it was?

I eventually realized I needed help. I ordered every book on eating disorders and binge eating, and everything I could find that had to do with building a better relationship with food. I started working on changing my relationship with food and overcoming my behaviors. I ended my black-and-white thinking and stopped bingeing.

Now, I look back and think about how far I've come. I remember feeling so hopeless that food was controlling my life and wanting so badly to end this cycle of bingeing, but not being able to. For the past 12 years, I've learned to enjoy healthy food and feel in control of what I eat, and I've realized that I feel better when I'm eating healthily. I also have an occasional splurge once or twice a week, which I enjoy every bite of and never feel guilty about. I am happy in my own body, feeling good about myself, and feeling empowered that I've come so far in my relationship with food. If you are grappling with the same issues or have struggled with them in the past, I hope to give

you the same sense of empowerment and confidence in your body.

Why am I telling you all this? Because I'm sure many of you can relate to my story. Maybe you never had an eating disorder, but you may have found yourself bingeing on foods, checking out from the stress of life. Or maybe you constantly go on diets and come off diets, losing weight and gaining it all back, over and over again. Most women have some kind of dysfunctional relationship with food. I tell you this because I no longer struggle with any of this. I see women struggling with food every day at my gym, and most of them think I have no idea what it's like, that it must be easy for me because I'm a "fitness female." How wrong they are! This did not come easily for me. I have worked very hard to build a healthy relationship with food and to stop beating myself up. I want to help you make that same mindset change and stop letting food control you and your happiness. Becoming a fit female is about being in control of who you are, what you eat, and how you feel. I'm telling you my story to give you hope and to inspire you to tackle your own relationship with food.

This book is not about overcoming eating disorders, but more about building a healthy relationship with food, fueling your fit female body, and feeling good about yourself and the choices you make every day. It's about knowing exactly how to find a balance between enjoying life and maintaining a fit, healthy, and sexy body. *(If you struggle with an eating disorder, you should seek the help of a professional.)* As you get into the workouts and are challenging your body to lift more weight, do more pushups, and push your intensity out of your comfort zone, you'll need to fuel yourself with healthy foods. Thinking of food as fuel for your fit female body will come, and you'll no longer struggle with the ups and downs of yo-yo dieting. You will be in control, instead of food controlling you.

Strategies for Overcoming a Destructive Relationship with Food

1. If you are a stress eater and you binge when you're under stress, start to keep a journal and write down your thoughts immediately following a binge. Start to recognize what emotions you have when you find yourself in the middle of a box of cookies. The goal initially is to binge less and less often and to start to understand what triggered you to do it. Eventually, instead of binge-ing, write in the journal first.

2. Eliminate all black-and-white thinking. You can have a splurge and not feel guilty about it. Really! Most women make the mistake of eating something that they know they shouldn't

and then feeling horrible about it. They beat themselves up, which then leads to their continuing to blow their diet because they figure they already screwed up—they may as well blow their diet some more. They feel like they've failed and it's no use because they have no willpower, so why even try? Sound familiar? Instead, choose your splurges wisely, but when you do decide to eat something you know you shouldn't, enjoy it fully and get back on track with your next meal. *You have not blown anything.* Stop beating yourself up! You won't eat enough to gain even a pound of fat. You would have to eat 3,500 extra

Fit Female Visual Tool

If you had a flat tire on your car that caused you to pull off the road, delaying you from getting where you want to go, would you (a) fix the tire and get back on the road or (b) go around and flatten all the other tires, making absolutely sure you would *never* get to your intended destination? I imagine you said (a), you would fix the tire and get back on the road. Well, then why is it so common for a female to blow her diet on one meal, eating something she shouldn't, but then, instead of getting back on track with her next meal and getting back on the road, go on to blow the whole day, the whole weekend, the whole week? This is blown tire syndrome: You blew one tire; you might as well blow them all! Not too logical, huh? Next time you blow a tire, fix it with the next meal and get back on the road to where you want to go!

calories beyond what you normally burn to gain a pound of fat—this would be very hard to do. If you get back on track, your body will burn even more because of the boost you gave your metabolism. Don't feel guilty about a splurge ever again. And keep in mind that a splurge is different from a binge. The goal is to end bingeing forever if you struggle with it. The 90% rule I talk about in the nutrition chapter gives you the freedom to have a splurge guilt free. Plan on having your 10 percent to splurge, and do not feel guilty. Allowing yourself this freedom will get you out of this black-and-white thinking.

3. Start to associate pigging out with the bloated, lethargic feeling you have afterward. Tune in to the way you feel and really connect in your head that when you eat that way, you don't feel good. At the same time, start to associate feeling full of energy and vitality and feeling good about yourself with eating healthy foods. Really connect with how these foods make you feel. This is a concept personal development coach Anthony Robbins talks about in his book *Awaken the Giant Within*. Basically, you work on associating more pain with the habits you want to get rid of and more pleasure with the habits you're working on creating. This pain-pleasure connection is extremely powerful in changing your behaviors over the long term.

4. Figure out what your trigger foods are. Certain foods will be your trigger to binge. Remember how we talked about having strategies? Having a strategy of not eating your trigger foods is extremely effective while you are working on your relationship with food. My trigger food used to be yogurt-covered pretzels. When I was stressed or emotional, I would get a big bag of yogurt-covered pretzels and start my binge, checking out from whatever was bothering me. Since I have made the breakthrough and overcome my destructive eating habits, I no longer even want yogurt-covered pretzels ever, because I have connected a bloated, lethargic, negative feeling to eating them. Realize what your trigger food is—usually it has that addictive substance sugar as an ingredient—and eliminate it from your environment. Food is a drug, especially sugar, and can absolutely be addictive. The highs and lows are very similar to the highs and lows addicts feel on drugs. Bingeing will give you a temporary high, escaping from reality, and then, *crash,* your blood sugar is in the gutter and you go into a sugar coma and need another fix. The hardest part is that food isn't something you can eliminate from your life—you have to eat.

By using the above strategies and following the nutrition principles to achieve a stable blood sugar, you can have a healthy relationship with food and become the fit and fabulous female you've always wanted to become. End the self-destructive cycle, end the addiction, end the unconscious eating and obsessive behaviors—you are fit and fabulous and deserve more!

It's time to fuel your fabulous body.

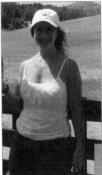

▲
Tiffany before

►
Tiffany as a fit female after losing 10 pounds of fat and gaining strength and definition.

FIT FEMALE *Real Life Story*

My story is really about taking everything I've learned through the years (including my calorie- and weight-obsessed upbringing by both parents and grandparents) and letting it go. I've learned it's not about how little you can eat and how much you can exercise. It's about balance, eating healthily to feel good (it's true!), and rebuilding self-confidence. It's about knowing that I don't need perfection and minimizing my own perfectionist tendencies. And it's about treating myself well so that I am happy and content with how I feel and look—not trying to fit some definition of what I should look like. I don't need to be the best. I need to be happy with my body and the strength and power it gives me to live the life I want.

This journey has definitely pulled me from the worst I've felt about myself, and transformed me into a person who is unwilling to put up with what she doesn't want—including a job that stressed me out and a body I wasn't treating well. Although I've always exercised and eaten well, I have battled with food as a soothing agent. Now I'm beginning to see myself differently. My legs are strong, my butt is lifted (yay!), and I'm toning my entire upper body. It's not about being a certain weight anymore—it's about being toned and feeling like I can conquer the world. ✦

Chapter 6

Hormones,
Schmormones . . .

Cramps . . . bloating . . . fat days . . . crying for no reason . . . it's all part of being a woman! Isn't it fabulous being a girl?

Recently I had a client say to me, "I was having the worst cravings all weekend, and I didn't give in. I was so proud of myself! But I got on the scale today and I gained two pounds! I'm quitting! I'm frustrated!" What we ended up figuring out was that the reason she was having these cravings was that she was having PMS. Her weight was probably up two pounds because she was holding some water. Most women retain a couple of pounds of water right before their periods. And of course, she was a little grumpy (not that we females will ever admit we're grumpy because our period is about to start). By the end of the week, she had lost the 2 pounds plus another pound, and she felt fabulous and focused again.

As you are becoming a fit female, you'll get in tune with your body and learn what works and what doesn't, and how your body responds to the fluctuations in hormones at different times of the month. You'll become aware of your cycle and how your body changes over the month—when you hold water, when you feel your best, when to push yourself in the gym (and when to give yourself a break), and how to feel fabulous all month long. Not all women are affected by the hormonal ups and downs that happen during their cycle. But some women are extremely sensitive, especially during that week when our "friend" comes to visit, to having extreme highs and lows with symptoms of PMS, including bloating, mood swings (not that we'll ever admit it), and cravings. These peaks and valleys can be very closely related to your nutrition and stress levels. Following the principles in this book should make you much less susceptible to the dramatic fluctuations in your hormones and symptoms.

The question is, should your training and nutrition change with your cycle? Getting in tune with your own cycle, which can vary but on average should be about 28 days long (although it may be as short as 18 days or as long as 40 days), is part of becoming a fit female. Many busy women don't pay close enough attention to their cycles. It's good to mark in your journal when you get your period so you can start to become familiar with your cycle, when to expect your period to arrive, and how to plan your training and nutrition around

it. There are a few things to keep in mind when it comes to your training, diet, and periods.

PERIOD WEEK (days one through five) Day one of your reproductive cycle is the first day of your period. During these four or five days of your menstrual cycle, you may have cramps and not feel 100 percent, but overall you should try to work out to decrease your symptoms. Your serotonin is lower at this time of the month, which may make you feel down in the dumps; but exercise boosts serotonin naturally, so get to the gym even if you don't feel like it. As the week progresses, your hormones should stabilize. In research, there have been conflicting reports, but more than one study has shown that exercise felt harder the week before and the week of women's periods because of increased levels of progesterone and decreased levels of serotonin, both of which have been linked to mood swings. I can tell you from subjective reports that most women don't feel optimal at this point in their cycles. You may find that your workouts feel harder than usual and that you're more tired, feeling drained of energy. Along with battling fatigue, you may also feel achy. Don't beat yourself up if you don't set a personal best this week. Just get in and get it done. By the end of this week, your hormones will level off, you'll start to feel good, and your cravings will disappear. Start to gear up for the next two weeks when you should be able to really push yourself in the gym.

Take advantage and burn more fat. The good news is that during the week before and the week of your period, your body does use fat for fuel more efficiently. I learned about this from Eric Serrano, M.D., and it was shown in a research study that examined the regulation of exercise carbohydrate metabolism by estrogen and progesterone in women. Problem is, your body knows this (our bodies are so smart), and with the decrease in serotonin during this time of the month, you will crave carbohydrates to give your body something other than fat to burn. Do your best to avoid giving in to your cravings, knowing that you'll actually burn more fat if you keep the carbs down at this time. This is a great reason not to miss your workouts—you'll burn more fat this week. More than once I have taken advantage of this with clients and encouraged them to stay superfocused the week before and the week of their period to break through a plateau or to dial it in for an event, and have seen it work to drop more fat than usual this time of the month. Use it to your advantage!

OPTIMAL HORMONES (days 6 through 20) The day after your period ends, get focused and take advantage of your hormones being optimal for your best performance in the gym. These two weeks in your cycle are the best time to dig deep and push yourself with your workouts. You should bump up your volume, your intensity should be high, and you should be using more weight. Challenge yourself by putting an all-out effort into every weight you lift and every interval you do. You should feel your best, because your hormones are the most

stable at this time of the month. Some women may start to feel PMS symptoms as early as day 14, when you will have a surge in estrogen during ovulation, but most women don't have symptoms until about day 21 or later. Again, the stages can vary dramatically from woman to woman, so it's important to get familiar with your own cycle. Overall, no excuses these two weeks to not challenge yourself in the gym to eke out as many reps as you possibly can! Stick to the Fit Female Credo Secret #4: Train hard or go home! Your cravings should also disappear, leaving you motivated to fuel your body with healthy foods.

PMS WEEK (days 21 through 28) As discussed above, PMS symptoms can start as early as day 14. If you are one of those women who have two weeks of PMS (you poor thing), there is hope! You should notice a difference when you start to get your blood sugar and stress levels stable; your hormones will also be more stable, with fewer highs and lows. Usually it's on days 21 through 28 that you don't feel your best with symptoms of PMS, including bloating, headaches, fatigue, cramping, sore breasts, body aches, and uncontrollable cravings. And of course most likely a huge pimple that just sprouted up on your face overnight to make you feel even better. You may gain some bloat, usually three to five pounds, which makes you feel even worse, but remember that it is temporary. It is not a reason to get frustrated and quit! It's easy to come up with an excuse or two not to work out at this time of the month, but don't rationalize putting off your workout, even though you're not feeling fabulous. Instead, get your workout done—you'll feel better! Research has shown that serotonin is lower and blood sugar levels, breathing rates, and body temperature all vary at this time of the month, but this is still not an excuse to skip your workout. This last week of your cycle, you may not feel as motivated to train, and injury risk is higher because of joint laxity and lack of focus. Keep this in mind and plan your training accordingly. If you get sore breasts, wear a supportive sports bra to keep the "girls" from bouncing. If you don't have one supportive enough, I give you permission to replace any of the hopping and jumping exercises for stationary squats if your breasts are too sore this week. I know how uncomfortable that can be, and it's enough to make you not want to work out. I can usually tell when a client is having PMS when she starts hopping on her warmup, because she immediately crosses her arms over her chest to hold everything still. This is fine, too. The programs in this book are in four-week phases, creating what we call a deloading week every fourth week, which is when you start a new program. Try to plan your training so that this week, days 21 through 28 of your cycle, lands on your first week of a new program, the deloading week. Again, some

WEEK 1

Start a New Program

1–2 sets only, lighter weights

learn new exercises

Okay to change jumps and hops to stationary

Body will use fat for fuel more efficiently— Stay focused!

Progesterone high, Serotonin Low

Cravings, bloat, cramps, sore breasts … hang in there!

PMS Week (days 21 to 28)

WEEK 2

Second Week on Program

Familiar with exercises, increase volume to 2–3 sets

Bump up your weights 10% on 2–3 exercises (not all of them)

Period Week (days 1 to 5)

WEEK 3

Third Week on Program

Increase your loads

Boost your intensity

Challenge yourself!

Bump up the weight again on 2–3 exercises (not all of them!)

WEEK 4

Last Week on Program

Time to get everything out of the workout! All-out effort!

Going for maximum demand on your body to get it to change

Use weights that you may not get every rep on every exercise (keeping your form, of course!)

Day 14–Ovulation

Surge in estrogen, Body temp increases, may be some weight gain

Hormones most stable

2 Weeks—Optimal Hormone Weeks (days 6 to 20)

WEEK 5 (Week 1 on new program)

Start a New Program

1–2 sets only, lighter weights

learn new exercises

Okay to change jumps and hops to stationary

Notice: Your intensity is lower, but is still a step up from 4 weeks ago

Body will use fat for fuel more efficiently

Progesterone high, Serotonin low

Cravings, bloat, cramps, sore breasts

PMS Week (days 21 to 28)

exercise will boost your serotonin and you'll burn more fat, so get to the gym even if you don't feel like it. Also, this boost in serotonin from your workout will help with your cravings. Just be cautious and listen to your body if something doesn't feel quite right.

The graph on page 71 is an example of how to plan your training. Your body may have a different cycle, so you may need to make adjustments as necessary. We'll cover more about planning your training in Chapter 10, Fit Female Workout Manifesto.

Something to look forward to: As you lose body fat and start living the lifestyle of a fit female, you'll have fewer dramatic symptoms of PMS and the highs and lows discussed above. This was demonstrated in a research study that showed that menstrual symptoms diminished significantly after women followed a physical training program. Having higher body fat can change your hormones quite a bit—especially estrogen, which is one of the main culprits behind all your symptoms. As you're losing fat, you may notice your periods becoming more regular and your PMS not being as extreme, and this is all because your hormones are stabilizing. Also, as your blood sugar and stress levels become stable, the symptoms will lessen.

I have experienced this myself. I've never really had severe symptoms of PMS or cramps (except maybe getting a little moody). But when I was in my "busting-out-of-my-fat-clothes" body, I experienced cramps for the

WHAT ABOUT THE PILL?

Nowadays, many women between the ages of 18 and 35 use some form of birth control. By using the Pill, you are adding a hormone to your body, and it can affect your progress in your efforts to reshape your body. The hormone you're adding is usually estrogen, which is the hormone that makes a woman a woman and gives us our baby-bearing hips. Everyone is different and is affected differently. However, the Pill is not an excuse not to become a fit female. Don't let yourself off the hook by saying, "Since I'm on the Pill, I'll never get as lean as I want to." There are so many different options now when it comes to birth control. As you get in tune with your body, be proactive about what you put into it. Talk to your doctor about the best option for you. If you notice that you're gaining weight on one pill, switch to a different one. Try one that's lower in estrogen or ask your doctor about switching to an IUD. Being a fit female is all about taking control of your own body and knowing what's best for you. Consult your doctor to determine what will work best for your body.

first time in my life and remember being curled up on the couch holding my stomach, understanding for the first time why women complain of cramps. Since making my breakthrough to achieve my fit female body, having stable blood sugar and hormones, I am back to experiencing minimal ups and downs during my cycle and never having cramps . . . but I do still get the occasional period pimple.

Following are a few tricks of the fit female trade to keep you feeling fabulous all month long.

HOW TO DEAL WITH SOME OF THE "NOT-SO-FIT-FEMALE" MOMENTS YOU MAY EXPERIENCE AS A WOMAN

Cravings Everything is going swimmingly. You're sticking to your plan and feeling good about yourself, and then . . . there it is . . . *that* time of the month. What is it about that time of the month that makes you crave stuff you haven't craved all month? Why do you start to lose your focus when it comes to sticking to your nutrition? Why do you just want to eat chocolate or carbohydrates? What makes you start to feel bloated, holding more water than usual, leading to "fat days" and feeling sorry for yourself? This is when you rationalize that you need to splurge more than your allotted 10 percent (which I'll explain in the nutrition chapter) because "I'm fat anyway. I may as well eat what I want this week. Who cares?" Then you feel worse about yourself, and the cycle continues. It might just be me, but I have a hunch that many of you reading this book have experienced this.

These cravings are physiological and have to do with your hormones, not your lack of self-control. The key is heading into this time of the month with the knowledge that you are in control and you will not let your hormones get the best of you. If you can keep your focus and stick to the nutrition rules 90 percent of the time this week, you'll find that you will actually lose more fat during this time of the month. That's right. During the week before and the week of your period, your body burns fat more efficiently, as I discussed earlier. Your level of serotonin (a "feel-good" hormone) drops, and your body craves carbs—it doesn't want you to burn fat. Fight the cravings and you can actually lose more. Also, do not skip your workout. Working out will give you a natural serotonin boost, helping to decrease the cravings.

You work hard all month to look and feel great—you don't have to feel fat and defeated for a week every month. Stay focused.

Bloating. If you have a tendency to get really bloated, follow these steps.

Drink extra water. As you're drinking water, your body will be less likely to hold on to water. Drinking more water will signal your kidneys to increase the hormones that tell your body to release water (making you pee). Keep the water coming in so your body will flush it out. You know you're properly hydrated when your urine is practically colorless.

Watch your sodium. If you stick to fresh foods, your sodium will automatically be lower. Be careful of eating out, having Chinese takeout, or eating anything packaged. Most of these foods contain extra sodium as a preservative.

Use natural diuretics such as vitamin C (take one to three grams a day), dandelion root, and asparagus. Also squeeze lemon in your water.

Keep starchy carbohydrates low. Stick to protein, fruits, and veggies to keep from holding water. Starchy carbs hold water and will increase your bloatedness.

Grumpiness. If you're following the Fit Female Nutrition Rules, your blood sugar should be stable, which will help keep your mood stable. Don't skip a meal and let your blood sugar crash. Be sure to eat protein at every meal. Keeping your blood sugar stable should help keep you from having mood swings. And above all, do not get to the state of total starvation! This could be disastrous. Don't mess with a hungry woman who is having PMS.

Cramps. Believe it or not, getting to the gym or at least going for a walk will help you battle painful cramps. I know you just want to curl up on the couch and feel sorry for yourself, but if you get out and move, you'll feel better! Cramps are basically a spasm of the uterine wall as it's shedding its lining. Doing some exercise can usually help calm it down. As you get into a regular routine of exercise and eating right, the cramps should become less severe. This has been my experience with my clients and myself.

Absence of periods. If you do not have periods—and you're not pregnant—this is not a good thing. This is actually a very dangerous situation. Not having a period is a sign that your body is not operating optimally. Your hormones are off kilter, and you need to listen to what your body is trying to say to you. A lapse in periods usually happens when your tub of stress is very full (see Secret #13 in the Fit Female Credo) and your body is telling you it can't take any more. Either life has given you too much stress or this could be a sign that you are overtraining (doing too much exercise). Or it could be that your body fat is so low that your body can't produce the hormones you need in order to have a regular cycle.

You need to get your body back to normal. Stop overtraining and take a day off. Take some time to relax (cortisol reduction time) and listen to your body. It is not healthy not to have periods. Everybody is different, but if the symptom is not addressed, usually the next sign is adrenal fatigue or depression, which can be very serious.

One of my clients was a 27-year-old female who, when I met her, was not having periods and hadn't had one for three years. She thought it was cool and wasn't worried about it. But as soon as she told me, I knew we had to address it. Turns out she was extremely overtrained and had some stressful events going on in her life, and her body needed a break! She was a cardio queen when I met her, taking five or six aerobics classes a week, going for a run a couple of days a week, and maybe hopping on an elliptical for 30 minutes to burn some extra calories. Her body fat hadn't changed despite all this exercise, so she just kept adding more. When she hired me to be her trainer, I made her stop all the cardio she was doing and take up strength training two or three days a week, with rest days on days in between, to get her system back to normal. She thought I was nuts but luckily trusted me enough to give it a try. Her body started to change before our eyes, developing abs that she'd never had before, and the day she got her period, you would have thought she was a teenager having her period for the first time. She called me immediately, and we were both so excited. I was so proud of her for getting her period! Kind of strange, but it was exciting because it meant her body was now back to normal and was operating optimally.

Throughout this journey, you are going to become so in tune with your body. As you lose body fat and gain muscle, your hormones will stabilize, and you'll find that your cycle may change, usually for the better. The hormonal fluctuations that make us women so unpredictable should not be nearly as bad. Hopefully you can get rid of the "period clothes" for good.

Low sex drive. We women are complex creatures, and our desire for sex is based on the interaction of a number of different variables, including how good we feel about ourselves. One of the main reasons women avoid sex is because of poor body image. We all know that when were feeling good about our bodies, we tend to be in the mood more often. Following the Fit Female Credo, nutrition rules, and workout program will lead to feeling better about yourself, improving your self-esteem, and having a new confidence in your body that will lead to a boost in your sex drive. Low sex drive can also stem from a decrease in testosterone, the hormone that increases sex drive in both men and women. Strength training can help give your testosterone levels a boost, which in turn will give your sex drive a boost. Don't worry, you'll never get enough testosterone to start looking like a man, but you can get enough of a boost to notice an uptick in your sex drive and improved fat burning. A natural rise in testosterone is a very good thing.

Chapter 7

At the Starting Line

You've set your goals, done your visualization, taken the Fit Female Credo to heart, and you're ready to get started!

Where are you now? What is your starting point for your journey to reinvent yourself as a fit female?

When beginning a program, you should get the following progress indicators on record. Have each of these in your toolbox to check yourself throughout your journey. I am all about tuning in to how you feel and look, but you also need indicators to tell you whether you're on track. This will help you determine whether you need to change something.

The most accurate and important measurement is a pair of what I call thermometer jeans.

✦ **Thermometer jeans.** Thermometer jeans tell you if you are getting closer to being HOT! And they tell you when you *are* HOT! And of course, most important, when you reach the point of maintaining your fit female body, they tell you when you're NOT! Remember, your goal is to be the BITCH in your thermometer jeans! BITCH = Be Inspiring, Totally Confident, and HOT! Once you've decided that you want to be fit and fabulous, buy a pair of jeans that you want to fit into or pull out that pair that's been hiding in the back of your closet. Whatever size you want to be in your fit body, have those jeans on hand. I recommend starting with a pair about two sizes too small. Keep them out where you can see them every day and try them on every couple of weeks. You might start off not even being able to pull the jeans over your thighs. A few weeks later, you'll be able to pull them up over your thighs, but they might get stuck on your hips. Eventually, you'll have them on, but there will be no way you can zip or button them. Then, lo and behold, the button will touch the hole and you'll be able to fasten it, but they'll still be so tight you would *never* wear them in public. Then at last they will be on, zipped, and fitting you pretty well. Soon enough, they'll fit you just right, when you are looking HOT and have become the BITCH!

These are now your thermometer jeans.

They tell you exactly where you are. They don't lie. These are the jeans that will tell you when you are straying from your fit female lifestyle too much and need to get back on track. They are the best measurement you have.

To weigh or not to weigh? The reason I like thermometer jeans is that this is *not a weight-loss program.* This is a completely REINVENT your body program! You will gain muscle while you lose fat, and the number on the scale might not budge as much as you might like it to. If you have some ideal weight that you think is where you need to be—*forget it!* Do not get stuck on a number. Instead, focus on what size jeans you want to be in and how you want to look.

One of my clients said to me, "I feel so great! I've lost two pants sizes and have gone from a size 14 to a size 10, but my weight hasn't budged, and I'm getting frustrated. My ultimate goal is to get into a size 6! But above all, I *have* to lose weight!" Do you see how hard my job is as a coach? She had gone from a size 14 to a size 10, but instead of being happy and enjoying her new body, she was frustrated that her weight had not come down. So I said to her, "What if you get down to a size 6, but your weight doesn't change and stays exactly where it is? Will you be happy?" "Absolutely not!" she shrieked. "I have to lose weight! I don't care if I am in a size 6 if my weight hasn't gone down!" So I asked her,

"Then you would rather stay in a size 10 and have your weight drop 10 pounds?" She said, "Yes, I want to lose the weight! I need to be in the 130s!" She could not comprehend what I was talking about. She very well may get down to a size 6, and her weight may not change much, but *who cares?* Nobody ever has to know your weight, but they will know that you are looking *hot* in your new size 6 jeans!

THE FAT-SUCKING MACHINE

If we had a magic fat-loss machine—a little booth that you stepped into and pushed a button, and you came out looking *exactly* how you've always dreamed of looking and feeling: the exact dress or pants size you want, with the definition and muscle tone you want, at the body fat percentage you want, with abs you can see (if that's what you're aiming for)—would you be interested? Of course you would! But what if the side effects of the fat-loss machine were that it increased bone density and muscle density by 100 percent? So, while you looked and felt better than you've ever felt before, the scale would read 50 pounds higher than it ever has. So, for example, a 150-pound woman would come out looking *amazing* but weighing 200 pounds. Would that number on the scale make you not want the other results? Now, what if the machine did the reverse—you'd look exactly the same as you always have, but you'd weigh 50 pounds less? Would you be happy with that? Probably not, right? Just understand that how you look and feel and how much you weigh are not necessarily related at all. If you add 10 pounds of muscle and lose 10 pounds of fat, you're going to look as if you lost *at least* 20 pounds. But the scale won't move. Don't focus on the scale. Focus on how you feel, how your clothes fit, and all the compliments you're getting! (Inspired by an article by Chris Shugart)

◆ **The Scale** Use the scale as *one* of your indicators, but do not misuse it. Understand that it is not the whole picture. The best time to weigh yourself is first thing in the morning, before you eat or drink anything, and it's best to use the same scale every time you reevaluate. The scale can be useful if it's used correctly. Do not let the scale tell you what kind of day you'll have today. If you find yourself getting on the scale and it ruins your entire day because it doesn't display the number you're looking for, *do not* get on the scale anymore. Do not empower a metal inanimate object to have that much control over your mood and what kind of day you'll have. It is just *one* measurement of your progress and will give you only *one* piece of the puzzle. Use it as information: When your weight is up, ask yourself, have I gained strength in the gym? Did I eat something with more sodium, or maybe it's the week before my period? The scale can be a very useful tool to help you get to know your body and how it responds to different foods and fluctuations at different times of the month. A fit female is in tune with her body. I'm not against checking your weight to see if you're moving in one direction or the other, but it is not the whole story. You cannot rely on weight as your only feedback on whether you're becoming fit. The reason is that you are changing your entire body composition, adding muscle and losing fat, so your body will be made up differently. This will not always be reflected on a scale. Most fit females you meet weigh a lot more than they appear to because they have muscle. Again, do not obsess about a number on the scale or "losing weight." You can do a starvation diet and lose weight, but your body will just look like a smaller version of your same self. That is not what this book is about.

This book is about completely reinventing your body—what it's made up of and how it looks—and increasing your metabolism to make it easy to keep your fit body when you get there. Since you'll be lifting weights and getting stronger, when your weight does drop, you'll know that what you've lost is pure body fat, because, if anything, you'll have gained muscle. So when the scale does go down a pound or two, you can call it a progress indicator, because you'll have been increasing your strength in the gym, so you'll know any weight you've lost is pure fat. You will be losing only fat during this program, no muscle. While reinventing your body, you'll be gaining muscle, and every pound you lose will be from pure fat. This is why your weight won't change as much as if this were just a weight-loss program. Keep in mind that when you do lose a pound of fat, it's equivalent to four sticks of butter off your body! That's a lot when it's pure fat coming off. I have had clients say, "I only lost a pound this week." What do you mean, "only a pound"? It's a pound of fat—4 sticks of butter—*gone!* That is a lot!

IMPORTANT: The number on the scale going down is a good thing, as long as you are getting stronger in the gym and building strength and muscle. Building strength and muscle means you're losing pure fat. The scale going up or staying the same *is not a bad thing* if other indicators are telling you your body is changing for the better, gaining muscle, changing shape, and so on. Got it?

◆ **Body fat calipers.** If you have access to a professional who can use body fat calipers to tell you your body fat, this can be a helpful measurement to have. Have the same person take it every time. Monitoring your body fat percentage will get your focus off the scale and on losing fat and gaining muscle. That's the ultimate goal in becoming a fit female. You can also use a bioimpedance machine, but know that with these machines your measurement may be affected by hydration, time of day, time of the month, and other factors. As a woman, you want to aim for between 18 and 22 percent body fat to achieve a lean, athletic look, but each person is different, so this number can vary. Usually, I find women are happy around 18–20 percent body fat.

Again, none of these measurements are the be-all and end-all, anyway. That's why it's good to have multiple indicators. Each of them is feedback on your progress. If your weight hasn't changed, but your thermometer jeans feel a tad looser and your body fat has gone down some, you're making progress! Or maybe your weight dropped two pounds but your body fat measurement says you gained a percentage point, yet you know you've gained strength in the gym. Those two pounds you lost must not be muscle, so you know you're making progress and haven't gained fat. The two pounds you lost could be water, in which case your body fat measurement can't tell the difference and will count it as muscle, giving you a higher body fat reading. As you lose fat, you'll also lose water, because fat cells are squishy and hold water. So we want that water gone. Overall, all these indicators are subject to interpretation, because none of them give you an exact picture of what's happening. However, taking them all regularly can give you helpful feedback on whether you're headed in the right direction.

✦ **Measuring tape.** Take a measurement of your bust, each arm, your waist, your hips, and each thigh. This won't tell you anything your thermometer jeans won't tell you, but again it's another reference point to see if you are making progress in your journey. The only problem with circumference measurements is that, like the scale, they may not tell you the whole story,

because if you don't have a butt but do have flab, as you start to build muscle in your butt, your hip measurement may go up. Make no mistake, this is a good thing, because you're building shape. Remember that great butt I talked about in the introduction? The one you could bounce a quarter off? That's what I'm talking about. Same with your legs—they'll build muscle that will firm them up and change their shape from flabby to firm. This is a good thing!

✦ **Photos.** Pictures are extremely powerful. Before you start the program, snap a few shots of yourself in a bathing suit or shorts and a half top. Put them away. If you're feeling discouraged midway through the program, pull out those original shots and take a few more to see how much you've changed. This is always eye opening, because seeing yourself in the mirror every day can be deceiving. It's hard to see the changes happening on a daily basis.

✦ **The mirror.** Then there's always the mirror test. The mirror is not your enemy. Sometimes it is hard to see the changes every day but you should check yourself out in the mirror to watch your body changing shape. You'll see definition where you didn't before and start to love the reflection staring back at you. Look in the mirror—do you like what you see? Do you look fabulous in your jeans?

"With hard work come results. The joy in life comes with working for and achieving something."

—Unknown

Check in with a progress indicator every week to keep yourself accountable and on track. The more reference points you have, the better. It's good not to just look at one thing when it comes to your progress, but instead have multiple ways to get feedback on how you're doing. This way, if your weight is not going down but your measurements are, you know you're making progress. Maybe the next week, your weight will drop but your thermometer jeans will still seem to fit the same, and you'll know you made some headway.

A client I was working with had lost 10 pounds the first five weeks we worked together and wanted to lose another 20 pounds. For a month, every week she got on the scale, and it said the exact same thing. Her body fat measurement was coming down and her clothes were fitting better, but the scale was not changing. Then suddenly, after three weeks—DROP! The scale showed she'd lost four pounds in one

Fit Female Tool

Realize that there is something I call the drop effect. Fat loss is never linear. I have never seen a client lose fat evenly week after week. It's always a big drop for a week or two. Then there's a plateau and then maybe another big drop, but sometimes the body gets stuck and plateaus at one spot for a period of time. This can be extremely frustrating for any woman. I tell my clients they need to stay focused and wait for the drop effect. The drop effect is the phenomenon that happens when your body is at a plateau and stays consistent week after week, until suddenly your body lets go and you drop anywhere from two to six pounds in one week. It may have something to do with fluid in the fat cells or your body not wanting to change; but in the real world, I know consistently I see women plateau for a period of time and then suddenly have a big drop when their fat loss catches up. This goes a long way in keeping you motivated to stick to the plan. You know that sooner or later the drop is coming, and even though you haven't lost any fat for a few weeks, your body will catch up. Just be patient and wait for the drop effect.

week. This is how it happened. So, really, she shed four pounds over four weeks, but it all came off in the fourth week. This can be frustrating and make you want to quit, so keep the drop effect in mind if your body seems to be stuck. Stay consistent and you will drop eventually.

Part 3

FUELING YOUR FIT FEMALE BODY

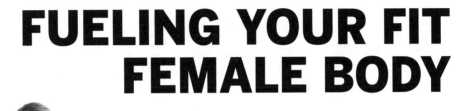

Chapter 8

Fuel to Be Fabulous

You Must Fuel Your Body to Give It What It Needs to Become Fabulous and Fit!

Eat more, burn more. To build this defined body you cannot starve yourself. This is also not about depriving yourself of social outings or enjoying an occasional cocktail because you are on such a strict diet. It is about figuring out the balance between eating the right foods to fuel your body and being able to live life to its fullest while feeling sexy, full of energy, and ready to take on anything. Most women have lost a bunch of weight and then put it back on again and press repeat. When you do a strict diet, you slow your metabolism down and you do not have energy to give your workouts 100 percent, much less live an active lifestyle. Your nutrition needs to fuel your new fit lifestyle. If you do not have enough of the right kind of "fuel in the tank," you will not get everything you can out of your training, nor will you have the building blocks to recover from your workouts. Just like the fitness training advice in this book, the nutrition advice is also based on solid research (it is not just my opinion),

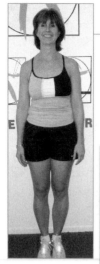

▲
Lesli before

**She lost
the last 10
pounds of fat
she had been
struggling
with.** ▶

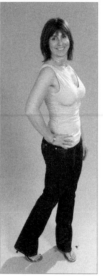

FIT FEMALE *Real Life Story*

I joined Results Fitness about 3½ years ago with the intention of losing those nagging 10 pounds that I had been struggling with and also to improve my overall fitness. I was able to accomplish those goals and so much more. I not only lost those unwanted pounds, I learned how to properly fuel my body so that I could get stronger and leaner. I learned that I was strong and have continued to get stronger with each day, month, and year that I work out. I have gained so much knowledge about nutrition, fat burning, weight training, and motivation. It may sound weird, but I truly love going to the gym and working out. I always leave feeling better than I did when I arrived. In fact, I look and feel better than I ever have before. I am so thankful for what I have learned on my journey and look forward to what I will continue to gain in the future. ✦

real world client results, and my experience with my own body. When you are putting the physical demands of training on your body and asking it to recover and repair itself, you have to give it the nutrients it needs to do so. The key is to eat more of the right things at the right time to boost your metabolism and give you energy. This allows you to burn more calories turning you into a fat-burning furnace which makes it easy to maintain your new body when you get there.

Before we get into specifics, I want you to keep two things in mind:

1. You cannot out-train a bad diet, so getting your nutrition figured out is extremely important. You don't want to work hard in the gym, spending time and energy only to go and screw it up by eating the wrong things. It isn't worth it! The food you eat needs to fuel your workouts. It is not as simple as burning off what you ate. "Gee, I ate a 500-calorie bowl of ice cream last night, I'll just get up early and do an hour of cardio and burn it off." Sorry girls, doesn't work. It is not as simple as that. When you get

your nutrition dialed in, the training programs work like magic.

2. The other thing to remember is that your goal is not to simply lose weight and be a smaller version of your same body. Rather, your goal is to completely change the way your body looks. If you simply wanted to lose weight, you could do that with a diet alone or with one of the fasts that are so popular (and dangerous) these days by eating less, losing muscle along with some fat, and end up looking exactly the same, only smaller. Your metabolism will have slowed down so it will be very hard to maintain. You would be what I call "skinny fat." Sure, you're skinny, but you are still flabby and don't look any better in a bathing suit, just smaller. This is not about simply losing weight, but changing your body into a transformed, toned, fit, sexy female.

So, what does a fit female eat? If you hate counting calories, you're going to love this: Counting calories is not necessary most of the time when you are working toward achieving your fit body. To obtain a fit, fabulous body, free of cellulite and belly fat, you must eliminate all processed foods—especially sugar. You are what you eat is very true and if you are feeding your body junk with no nutritional content, you can't expect to build a beautiful body. Until you have figured out what you should eat, you do not need to worry about calories, grams, or counting anything. Most of us girls have done enough calorie counting, fat gram counting, and carb counting to drive anyone crazy. Enough with the counting! Instead your focus should be on giving your body what it needs when it needs it, so you can have energy, burn fat, recover from your workouts, and boost your metabolism.

"Your appearance on the outside is a reflection of what is going on inside."

—UNKNOWN

A friend of mine and nutrition researcher, Mike Roussell, came up with what he calls the spectrum of nutritional habits, and I have found it really useful when working with my clients. The idea is to transition from a diet of what he calls "nutritional freestyling" or eating whatever, whenever, to being 90 percent compliant with proper food choices. You don't have to count every calorie and every morsel of food you put in your mouth to get the body you want. Of course, down the road after you have been following the basics, you may find that you have hit a plateau, or that you want to fine tune to reach a specific goal. That might be a case where you'll want to pay closer attention to your caloric intake. In most cases, however, I find that when people eliminate the junk food and start following the basic nutrition rules and "eating clean," their body morphs into a fit female body without having to count anything.

Where are you on the nutritional habits spectrum?

1. Nutritional Freestyling. This is where most people are most of their life. Eating whatever, whenever with no real plan or preparation. If this is where you are on this spectrum, you need to start moving down the spectrum to get a fit female body.

2. Proper Food Choices, Varying Compliance. This is where you know what you should eat and you eat it "most of the time." Do you remember, we talked about "most of the time" back in the Credo, Secret #16? However, what I find is that the average person who thinks they "eat pretty healthy" only eats what they should about 70 percent of the time. This is not enough to achieve the fit and fabulous body you want. I've had clients who say, "I am following what you're telling me most of the time, but my body isn't changing." That's because you are only following the basic nutrition principles 70 percent of the time, which may seem adequate, but isn't enough to change your body.

3. Proper Food Choices, 90 percent compliant. This is where you want to be to get your fit female body. Eat the right food choices 90 percent of the time and your body will transform. You do not have to count calories, but rather simply follow the rules laid out for you in the base phase in the pages to come and stick to them 90 percent of the time. This allows you 10 percent of your week to indulge and enjoy yourself without guilt.

4. Calorie/Portion Counting, Proper Food Choices, 90 percent compliant. This last spot on the spectrum is where we start counting calories. This is at the very end of the spectrum and it's really only necessary to go to this place when you have been 90% compliant and are ready to dial it in and fine tune if you've hit a plateau or if you're preparing for an event or specific goal. The majority of the time it is not necessary to count anything, so just relax and stop counting every gram, calorie and morsel you put in your mouth.

Determine where you are on the nutritional habits spectrum, and read on to figure out the plan to transition you from nutritional free-styling to a fit female who is 90 percent compliant! Or maybe you are already at number four above and are counting grams, calories, and every morsel of food but forgot about the basics. Let go of all of the counting and get back to basics. Start with the base phase and get the basics down first. There is no reason to drastically change your diet when you are getting started. Remember, you are becoming a fit female for life and building these habits for the long term.

Start by eating foods as close to their original source as possible, meaning fresh, unprocessed foods. We're talking about vegetables and fruits in particular. Additionally you will eliminate sugar, high fructose corn syrup, and highly processed foods, while you space out your meals throughout the day into smaller portions. As the old adage goes, if it has a bunch of ingredients you can't pronounce, don't eat it! If it grows from the ground or a tree, enjoy as much as you want. If it ran, flew, or swam, it is allowed. Unfortunately this approach runs counter to the typical western diet, which relies almost exclusively on large amounts of processed foods, processed meats full of nitrites and trans fats. This typical diet is why most women have cellulite, belly flab, and do not like the way they look. I have always believed that the way you look on the outside is a direct reflection of what is going on inside. Feed your body healthy, "clean" foods and your reflection will show a vibrant, healthy body! Have you heard the term "eating clean"? Eating clean is actually part of the lingo fit females and fit males have used for a long time to describe a diet free of junk food, sugar, high fructose corn syrup, trans fats, and any other processed food.

Being a fit female entails preparing and packing all of the foods your body needs for daily fuel, being conscious of what you are eating, and when and how often you decide to

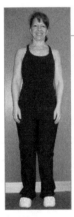

▲
Sharon before

She reinvented herself by losing 10 pounds of fat and gaining six-pack abs. ▶

FIT FEMALE *Real Life Story*

I've struggled with my weight since my early teenage years and tried many weight loss programs. In the past, I've had moderate success at weight loss for

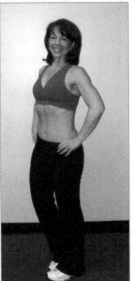

short periods of time, only to regain the weight and cause myself a lot of frustration and guilt. I joined Results Fitness in 2007 with a goal of weight loss. I wanted to lose weight in my hips and thighs because I've always carried my weight there. While I have lost weight, the best outcome by far has been the overall shape of my body. My body looks leaner and stronger and much more in proportion. I've also learned to think of food as fuel, rather than something dangerous for my body. I actually eat more food now than I ever have before, and I don't live with the guilt. I love my lean body and I plan to weight train for the rest of my life! ✦

#1 MISTAKES WOMEN MAKE WITH THEIR DIET THAT KEEP THEM FROM BECOMING FIT AND FABULOUS

1. **STARVING THEIR BODIES.** Why do so many women have it ingrained in their heads that they have to starve themselves to look the way they want? Is it because they get a sense of satisfaction when they skip a meal or only have sprouts or lettuce, thinking they have so much self-control? Maybe. But what those women should know is that they are starving their bodies right into a cycle of storing fat, losing muscle, and wreaking havoc on their metabolism. This is the last thing you should do if you want to look like a fit female. More often than not I hear this from my clients when I talk about their nutrition: "This is too much food! I can't eat all of this! How am I supposed to lose weight eating all of this food?" I tell them to give it a try and guess what? They become believers because their metabolisms increase and they burn fat! Picking up what I'm putting down? Do not starve yourself!

2. **ELIMINATING FAT.** Most of us girls have done it— counted our fat grams. I remember keeping track of every fat gram and not letting myself eat more than 15 fat grams a day. Dietary fat and body fat are two different substances. You don't eat fat and it gets turned into fat. That's not how it works. You must include good quality fats throughout the day. This is so important for your hormones, fat loss, and overall health. Increasing your Omega-3 intake (the fats found in fish, olive oil, avocado, nuts) has been shown to boost your body's fat burning ability. Do not be afraid of fat.

3. **ALL-OR-NOTHING THINKING.** Women tend to be very black and white, on or off. They are either on their diet super strict and focused, or they are OFF their diet and bingeing on foods they shouldn't be and beating themselves up over and over again. I see this all the time. It is either one or the other. If you are struggling with this, go back and read Chapter 5 again, especially Strategies for Overcoming a Destructive Relationship with Food.

4. **HAVING A FEAR OF CARBOHYDRATES.** Most carbohydrates are not the enemy. Certain kinds of carbohydrates are not an optimal fuel source for a fit female and you should avoid them or at least be mindful of when you have them. Fruits and vegetables are carbohydrates that you can have at any time during the day. Eaten with some protein, these produce picks are a perfect fit female food. Starches such as oatmeal, rice, and the other whole grains listed on the grocery list are perfect for breakfast or for the meal after your workout. Don't be afraid of these carbohydrates, especially post-workout. You need to refill your glycogen levels immediately following your workout. Eat your carbs—just the right kinds at the right times! Remember, it is the high sugar, highly processed carbs that you need to keep to a minimum.

5. **NOT PLANNING OR PREPARING.** Many women find it hard to put themselves first. Women are caregivers by nature and take care of everyone else. Problem is, when they don't take care of themselves they cannot give their best to everyone else. To be a fit female you have to take the time to plan and prepare your meals. You cannot leave it to chance. You don't become a fit female by chance. As the saying goes, Fail to plan, you can plan to fail! It won't take as long as you think to throw some healthy food into an ice chest each day. Give yourself 10 extra minutes a day to pack your food and plan your day.

splurge. It may seem like a lot of work at first, but what you will realize is that you feel better when you eat healthier foods. I know what you're thinking—*yeah, right . . . I could never give up my (insert your favorite food here).* Well, the good news is you don't have to. You can fit anything in as long as the majority of the time, you are willing to change the way you eat.

BASE PHASE FIT FEMALE NUTRITION RULES FOR LIFE

Eat breakfast within 15 minutes of waking up followed by a meal every 3–4 hours. You must keep fuel coming in all day to keep your blood sugar stable starting first thing in the morning. Your body is in a fasted state when you wake up because you have not eaten for 8–12 hours. Being in a fasted state is not optimal because it means your metabolism is in the gutter and you are not burning fat. A study released in June 2008, done at Virginia Commonwealth University, showed that women eating a large 600-calorie breakfast lost an average of 40 pounds over 8 months compared to a group who ate a lower calorie breakfast and only lost 9 pounds over the 8 months. The biggest key to this study was that the big breakfast eaters were able to maintain their weight loss while the small breakfast eaters started to put the pounds back on. In addition to having breakfast, to become a fit female you need to con-tinue fueling your metabolism every 3–4 hours. Again, not just something I came up with but has been shown in the research-

◆ In a study of meal frequency, it was shown that a group eating 6 meals per day lost more fat than a group eating 2 meals per day—despite calories being equal.

◆ A second study showed that irregular meal intake was associated with a lower thermic effect of feeding (calories burned as a result of the meal) than a regular meal pattern (6 meals per day) despite total meals per week being the same.

◆ And yet a third study showed that adults who were accustomed to eating 4 meals a day switched to 3 meals a day and gained body fat and weight despite calories remaining the same.

Also, skipping meals increases your likelihood of metabolic syndrome, which includes decreasing your good cholesterol, increasing your blood pressure, and worst of all increasing your belly fat. Why is this? Fasting decreases insulin sensitivity, which means your body becomes insulin resistant, or it has trouble removing sugar from the blood, leading to metabolic syndrome. Do not skip meals! Skipping meals can also lead to the **State of Total Starvation**. Avoid The State of Total Starvation at all costs!

State of Total Starvation: Occurs when you are so hungry, to the point of rationalizing eating anything. "It doesn't matter if it follows the rules or not, just give me food!" You start to check out, and are no longer what I call consciously eating or able to make an educated decision about a food choice. This state of mind causes you to be highly likely to overeat to the point of being completely stuffed. Unfortunately, soon after you indulge in whatever you could get across your lips first and your state of total starvation dissipates, you have feelings of remorse and disappointment. Maybe it's the feeling that you did not even want whatever it was you ate and that you wasted one of your splurges on it. Avoid the State of Total Starvation at all costs!

Do not go to the gym when you are running on empty. Have a small snack before you hit the weights. You cannot expect your body to perform when you have not given it some fuel. If you are training first thing in the morning, make yourself a shake and drink half before you start and finish it when you are done. There is no point in doing a workout on an empty stomach. You will not be able to push yourself to get the results you want if you don't start with some fuel in your tank.

WHERE IS YOUR BLOOD SUGAR?

Three Places Your Blood Sugar Can Be

LOW (in the gutter)—Your body is in a fasted, starving state and will not burn fat. It will actually store fat because it is in a panic that you are starving.

STABLE (burning fat)—To be a fit female you must figure out how to get your blood sugar stable and keep it there. The goal with the fit female nutrition rules is to get your blood sugar stable as soon as possible each day and keep it there all day long. When your blood sugar is stable, meaning not plummeting into the gutter, but not sky high, your body will be happiest and will burn fat and build muscle because it has everything it needs.

HIGH (in storage mode)—Your body has more sugar than it needs and is in storage mode. When your body has a surplus, it will store for later. The other problem with having your blood sugar high is that what goes up must come down, so as quickly as your blood sugar shot up it will plummet into the gutter very quickly.

Fuel Your Fat-Burning Furnace

Think of your metabolism as a fire. For a fire (your metabolism) to burn, you need to constantly be fueling it with new logs (food). As the logs go on the fire, the fire burns stronger, and gives off heat (burning calories). If you didn't fuel the fire, the fire would slowly burn out (stop burning calories) and then, as you notice the fire about to burn out (your hunger overtakes you in a state of total starvation), you dump on a bunch of logs (eat a HUGE, non-nutritious meal), and then the fire is suffocated and goes completely out (your metabolism is in the gutter). This is what most people do—they put their own fire out by either starving it or suffocating it. Instead, add fuel to the fire in small increments over time to keep it burning. Fuel your fire to burn fat and be fabulous!

1. Use protein shakes and bars. Sometimes you cannot prepare all 5-6 meals to bring with you for the day so you may need to grab something fast that you know contains the right amounts of nutrients you need. This is where protein bars and shakes come in handy. They make your life easier! They are really just food, but quick and easy food for when you are on the run. Protein bars need to be your back up plan, not your "everyday" plan. Real food is always a healthier choice. When is a protein bar acceptable? You should never miss a meal (because it will lead to a drop in your metabolism and breakdown of muscle tissue) so in an emergency you should always carry a protein bar with you. If you get stuck and it has been over three hours and you have not eaten and you are getting dangerously close to the *State of Total Starvation* (see above), then you are well prepared by having a bar in your purse to save the day and save your metabolism! Again, think of it as a backup plan but don't make protein bars part of your "everyday" plan. Instead, have yogurt, nuts, fruit and other real food snacks and save your bars for "in an emergency only." Most protein shakes are better quality than the protein bars. Many of the protein bars are loaded with sugar. If you have a choice, use a shake instead of a bar. Check the ingredients of either one and do not consume it if it contains anything that says

"hydrogenated," "partially hydrogenated," or any high fructose corn syrup.

2. Eat a mixture of high-quality protein at every meal. Protein contains amino acids, which are what your body needs to build muscle. Never eat carbohydrates alone. Why? Carbohydrates raise your blood sugar, some faster than others, telling your body to go into storage mode. Protein blunts this increase in your blood sugar, keeping you in a stable fat-burning mode. At every meal have a source of protein with a carbohydrate. Again, not just my opinion . . . A research study published in 2008 showed that adding eggs to your breakfast enhances weight loss, and another study showed that adding whey protein to the subjects' diet, resulted in a loss of 6.1 percent of their body fat mass which is a significant amount. And yet another study showed that lower carbohydrate, higher protein diets favorably affect body mass and body composition independent of how many calories they ate. It is important that you eat a protein with each meal to keep you in a fat burning state all day long. For your breakfast, lunch, and dinner, shoot for 4–6 ounces of protein which looks like the size of the palm of your hand. You do not need to get your scale out, just eyeball it. But be sure you are getting enough. In a later phase we will talk about using a scale, but for now just get the junk out and get the good stuff in.

3. Don't be afraid of red meat. Beef is a great source of protein and is the most highly absorbable iron you can get. Many women struggle with low iron levels, which will make you feel tired and fatigued, so beef is a good option once a week, especially if you're iron deficient. Try to get organic, grass-fed beef if possible.

4. Eat a fruit or vegetable at every meal and snack. A common mistake when women start to clean up their diet is to eliminate carbs, even the good ones. You can eat a lot more vegetables and fruits for the calories than you can starchy carbohydrates. Eating a vegetable or fruit at every meal will fill you up on the least amount of calories. You need to eat protein at every meal but you also need to eat a fruit or vegetable at every meal. Eating too much protein by itself will lead to an unhealthy environment in your body. Protein is very acidic, and if you are not eating your fruits and veggies to balance out that acidity, it creates an unhealthy situation. Plus, fruits and veggies provide your body with fiber, vitamins, minerals, antioxidants, and lots of good stuff. And they are generally lower glycemic, so they don't spike your blood sugar into storage mode like starchier carbs do. Eat a fruit or a vegetable at every meal. Once you get in this habit, it will become easy.

5. Eliminate all processed carbohydrates. Some carbohydrates will raise your blood sugar faster than others. You want to completely avoid the carbohydrates that will shoot your blood sugar straight into fat-storing mode; this includes processed foods such as breads, pasta, pastries, cereal, and sugar. Keep in mind, research showed that lower carbohydrate diets (namely lower processed starchy carbohydrates) equal greater fat loss. One study showed that at the *same* caloric intake, a reduced carbohydrate diet resulted in significantly greater fat loss (and participant retention) than a low-fat diet. Your carbohydrate sources should be primarily from fruits and vegetables, along with some whole grains such as rice and oatmeal.

6. Use healthy fats and oils freely. Don't be afraid of fats! You need fat. No more fat-free creamer, fat-free peanut butter, etc. Most fat-free products replace the fat with sugar. Read your labels. Healthy fats include avocado (my favorite), nuts, seeds, olive oil. Check out the grocery list in the next chapter, stock up on good fats, and incorporate them into your diet. People get confused and think that if they eat fat they will gain fat, but the two really are not connected to each other. Dietary fat is different from body fat. Dietary fat does not equal an increase in body fat . . . a diet full of processed junk food equals an increase in body fat. In fact, having omega-3 fats has been shown to decrease your body fat. Isn't that amazing, that eating fat will help you get rid of fat?

7. Eliminate caloric beverages and drink half your body weight in ounces of water everyday. Being dehydrated is a big "no-no" when it comes to achieving a fit and fabulous body. Dehydration takes away from your exercise performance which leads to decreased results, fatigue, and increased cortisol levels, your stress hormone that breaks down muscle tissue (BAD!). Also, if you do not drink enough water your body will hold on to water—aren't our bodies fascinating? Your pee should be clear. If your pee is not clear you are not drinking enough water. In a study done in 2008, women increased their water consumption to 1 liter a day and the researchers credited 5 pounds lost to the increase in water intake. Think of water as your fat flushing tool. If you have a diet soda habit, it is time to cut it out. Diet soda does nothing for your health. Diet soda is full of chemicals, artificial sweeteners, and ingredients whose long-term effects we don't truly know completely. You are better off without it. Stick with water. You can have tea and coffee in moderation. Drink mostly water throughout the day. You can squeeze some lemon, orange slices, or lime into it to give it flavor.

MY MORNING RENDEZVOUS WITH . . . JOE

I spend every morning with my cup of Joe . . . I love the smell, the taste, and the buzz of energy it gives me. As long as you stick to 1–2 cups a day, coffee can be a potent addition to a fat- burning plan and can be beneficial to simply get you going in the morning to work out. Moderate amounts of caffeine have been shown in the research to improve decision-making and reaction time, improve exercise performance by reducing the rate of muscle fatigue, and increase your body's ability to burn fat. Stick with black coffee with a small amount of cream or skim milk, skip the syrups and flavorings that add extra calories in the form of sugar. Caffeine does have diuretic effects, so be sure to drink plenty of water, but otherwise enjoy your cup of Joe! The key with caffeine is to use it in moderation and don't become dependent on it.

However, a better choice than a cup of "Joe" would be green tea

There is lots of good stuff in green tea that is hard to pronounce . . . catechin-polyphenols including one called Epigallocatechin 3-gallate (EGCG) which scientists believe is one of the active ingredients in green tea that helps people lose weight. We'll just call it "good stuff." British researchers found that this "good stuff" in green tea increased fat use by 17 percent during 30 minutes of exercise. It seems that when this "good stuff" interacts with caffeine it produces a fat-burning effect. Green tea can also lower cholesterol, increase calorie burning, and it contains antioxidants to protect your cells. It can also help to keep blood sugar and insulin levels stable, as shown in another study in 2006. Drink green tea instead of coffee in the morning or use a green tea supplement. It will help you to burn fat and be healthy! Occasionally I stray from "Joe" . . . for a cup of green tea . . . because it has more to offer me.

8. **Eat whole foods instead of bars and shakes whenever possible except for postworkout.** Consuming whole foods gives you more nutrition, more fiber, more nutrients, and has a higher thermic effect of food, which means you will burn more calories breaking down

whole food. Remember, save bars and shakes for your "backup" plan, not your "everyday" plan. Instead, pack a small ice chest of protein, fresh fruits, vegetables, nuts, yogurt and other good snacks. The only case when a shake is a better choice is postworkout when you need to get the nutrients in as quickly as possible.

9. Supplement with a multivitamin and omega-3 fish oils daily.

All of these rules . . . you're probably thinking, isn't there a magic pill I can take? Everyone wants the secret, magic fat-burning pill that will do all of the work for them. Sorry, girls, wish I knew of one. But the magic pill = Train Hard and Eat Healthy. There is no way around it, you have to put the work in. I know, not what you wanted to hear, sorry! But along with eating right and training hard, another important part of the fit female plan is supplementation. Supplements allow you to fill the gaps you might be missing with your nutrition. These are not magic pills, these are supplements, meaning they are meant to supplement a healthy nutrition and exercise plan. You should be using supplements as part of a healthy plan, but don't expect them to do the work *for* you.

FIT FEMALE DAILY SUPPLEMENT ARSENAL

10. Multivitamin/Mineral Every fit female needs to take a high-quality multivitamin/mineral supplement. Vitamins are your little helpers when it comes to making things happen with your body. They play many key roles in the body, including acting as cofactors and/or enzymes for certain reactions. This means they are absolutely necessary for certain reactions to happen including burning fat, making energy, and building muscle. Your health won't be optimal if you don't have enough of the right vitamins. Take a multivitamin with food every morning. This is your insurance policy ensuring you are getting everything you need.

Omega-3 or Fish Oils The special fats in fish, called omega-3 fatty acids, actually lower the level of unhealthy fats in the body by influencing the enzymes that synthesize fat and those that increase fat burning in the liver. A study, published in the *American Journal of Clinical Nutrition* in 2007, showed that supplementing with fish oil reduced body fat independent of exercise. Not only is fish oil beneficial for fat loss, but also for immune function, reducing inflammation, decreasing blood pressure, and reducing the risk for many other diseases such as cancer and cardiovascular disease. It is a good idea to take 3–6 grams of omega-3 fatty acids in supplemental form a day along with eating fish a couple of times a week to assure that you get enough omega-3 in your diet. Take them with food. Trick of the fit female trade: If you have trouble with them smelling fishy, stick them in the freezer.

11. Always drink a workout shake either during your workout or within 10 minutes of finishing your workout. Use a high-quality whey protein shake (with 20–30 grams of protein) mixed with fruit or other carbohydrate. Do not skip this step! This is so important I will discuss it again in Chapter 12, Recovery and Regeneration Rituals. Having a shake helps you get everything you can from your workout. It's crucial to replenish your body immediately after your workout with quick-releasing carbs and fats (a shake is best) to ensure optimal recovery. You must surround your workout with nutrition meaning you need to eat pre- and postworkout. The easiest and most useable source of nutrition is through a liquid protein/carbohydrate shake. A study published by John Berardi Ph.D. *et al.* in 2006 showed that having protein and carbohydrates together works best to replenish your body postworkout while other studies have shown that it increases protein synthesis. I recommend my clients start drinking their shake during the workout and finish it immediately after. The usual shake should be made up of blended whole fruits and whey protein powder. Having this shake during and postworkout will help repair and rebuild your body after a hard workout and is a mandatory supplement to your nutrition program. Whey protein has all of the amino acids your body needs to build muscle and repair after a workout. Whey protein is essential for building your fit female body.

12. **Keep a journal of what you are eating and stick to the rules 90% of the time. Plan to splurge 10% of the time.** A journal will keep you accountable and on track. To become fit and fabulous, you must keep track of what you are doing so you can look back and make changes if you need to. Eventually you can simplify this by using the grid I describe in the next chapter, but for the base phase jot everything down to keep you conscious of what you are eating and most importantly how often you are enjoying a splurge.

"I generally avoid temptation unless I can't resist."

—MAE WEST

Splurge: I like the word "splurge" because when you splurge you are treating yourself to something you really want. Whether it is a day at the spa, a new pair of expensive shoes, or your favorite decadent dessert, it always feels good. Everyone needs to splurge in life! The key is to splurge wisely and fully enjoy it. Do not feel bad about it. Do not beat yourself up when you decide to splurge. There is room to rebel in this plan. Enjoy every bite or every sip when you do! I think it is a good strategy to splurge outside of your house because it allows you to enjoy what you want and then leave it. If you splurge at home, you may find you end up with leftover ice cream in your fridge or leftover wine and guess what? You'll find yourself splurging again and again until you've exceeded your 10%. Don't think of your splurges as a "cheat" or feel guilty about them. Instead, enjoy every bite you take and know that you are allowed to splurge occasionally because it is the exception, not the norm. Just make sure your splurge(s) make up less than 10% of your meals each week.

Keep in mind, if you miss a meal or you

violate one of the rules above, including not having a fruit or veggie at a meal, you are choosing to splurge. In other words, don't blow your 10% all at once. It is just like shopping, you have a budget each week to shop with and you have to decide what will be worth splurging on and what is not worth it.

Remember, you have up to 3–4 splurges a week. And you don't have to use all four every week, but you also don't get to stockpile them up and use 16 in one week. It's not like rollover minutes on a cell phone plan, ladies!

The above rules are your nutrition rules for life.

FIT FEMALE *Real Life Success Story*

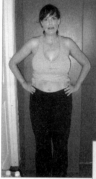

▲
Lori before

Lori lost 15 pounds of fat and 2 clothing sizes. ▶

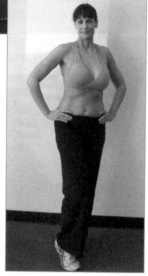

I can look at a photo album of myself over the past 20 years, and the photos where I am overweight and out of shape were also the times in my life when I did not have control of my life. Such a time was this past year when my life went spiraling out of control. Along with the spiral came the pounds. True, I had just had a baby; and true, I had just been through a traumatic relationship with an abusive alcoholic.

After going through days and weeks where I was so depressed I could barely get out of bed (only to care for my newborn, to eat, or to use the bathroom), I had finally had enough. I did what I always did when my life had tilted too far: I got back in shape.

I went back to see Rachel at Results (who welcomed me with open arms) and began my remake. I started out with baby steps: two times a week with a coach. Eventually I moved to three times and now have added a fourth day of interval/cardio. Believe me, it wasn't easy. Money was tight and what to do with my children was always an issue. But, where there is a will there is a way! Of course I added nutrition back into my life as well. I planned six small healthful meals a day and I stuck to it faithfully. I am happy to report that I lost 22 pounds of fat and look and feel fantastic. Not only did I physically get into shape, but mentally, emotionally, and spiritually followed like stepping stones. I urge you and anyone I know to begin within themselves, and everything else will follow—I guarantee it! ✦

Chapter 9

16-Week Fit Female Nutrition Action Plan

BASE PHASE: WEEKS ONE THROUGH FOUR—FIT AND FABULOUS!

Week one, it's time to clean it up! During this first four weeks, you'll focus on starting to "eat clean," as we discussed in the last chapter. This includes drinking plenty of water, fueling your body every couple of hours, eliminating the junk, and keeping a journal. This first four weeks is about building habits. The first few days will be the hardest, but once you get in your groove, it'll be smooth sailing. Remember Secret #2 from the Fit Female Credo: Get out of your comfort zone. Any time you make a change, it can be a little uncomfortable for a while until it becomes a habit.

"We've all heard the expression 'An apple a day keeps the doctor away.' Well, I've got a good question for you: What if it's true? Wouldn't that be easy to do—to eat an apple a day? Here's the problem: It's also easy not to do."

—JIM ROHN

The basic fit female nutrition rules are listed below. Go through each rule and check it off if you are already doing it. If you come across something you're not already doing, start today, and by the end of the first week you should already feel your body changing. I have seen people lose five to eight pounds the first week simply by drinking enough water.

The following rules are your rules for life. Once you create your fit female body and are where you want to be, you'll continue to eat following these rules so you can maintain your new shape. It's much harder to spur your body to change than it is to maintain once you are where you want to be. After you follow these rules for four weeks, we'll introduce some changes to keep your body from figuring it out. Your body will start to adapt to your nutrition plan, just as it adapts to your workouts, so to continue transforming yourself, you may need to change your approach along the way. Once you get to where you want to be, you'll be able to stick to these basic principles and keep your fit female body long term. As long as you're making progress, you don't need to change a thing; but if you start to plateau, it's time to tighten up the diet even more.

"Never eat anything in one sitting that you can't lift."

—MISS PIGGY

Base Phase

First things first: Eliminate the junk and stock up on healthy fuel! You cannot have a houseful of forbidden foods and expect success. Get rid of anything that's likely to trigger you to slip up. Everyone has trigger foods, and the last place they should be is in your house. That's right—throw out the bag of chips you've been working on! And that carton of ice cream that's been calling your name? Toss it out! Remember Fit Female Credo Secret #15: Don't rely on willpower. Have strategies.—Willpower isn't that strong. So you'll need to stock your house with everything you need to be successful and get in the habit of being prepared. The key to success is to prepare ahead of time. Do not leave your nutrition to chance. There is no excuse not to pack a small cooler and bring all the healthy food you need for the day with you everywhere you go! This is about building habits.

The following things need to be removed from your kitchen:

+ **All processed junk food.** Pretty much anything with more than a couple of ingredients or anything you cannot pronounce is processed and is not part of the fit female plan. This includes wheat products such as breads, crackers, chips, cereals, pasta, and bagels. Get them out!

Sugar. Check your food labels for the word *sugar*. It may also be disguised as fructose, glucose, or sucrose. Anything ending in *-ose* is a sugar. It may also be disguised as high fructose corn syrup. Check your ingredients. Even many of the processed peanut butters contain sugar and hydrogenated fats. Stick to all natural. For example, Skippy and Jif peanut butter ingredients look something like this:

Ingredients

Peanuts, Sugar, Partially Hydrogenated Vegetable Oil (Soybean), Fully Hydrogenated Vegetable Oils (Rapeseed and Soybean), Mono- and Diglycerides and Salt.

Natural peanut butter will have only peanuts and salt.

All calorie-containing beverages. No more soda and no more juice. Throw them out. I would rather you eat the fruit than drink the fruit. And absolutely no soda. And as for alcohol . . . Yes, the bottle of red wine that you were "only" drinking because of the antioxidants! More than one drink of alcohol per day increases your risk of metabolic syndrome, which means it increases your likelihood of gaining unsightly belly fat! You can enjoy a glass as part of your 10 percent weekly allotment of splurges (more on that later), but it's a good idea to get it out of the house to break your habit of having a nightly glass of wine.

Next you'll need to make a grocery trip and stock up on everything you'll need to be a fit female, so that you're not caught short and don't end up cheating in a weak moment when nothing else is available. Go through the following grocery list and highlight the stuff you like. Then hit the grocery store and fill that cart with fit female food!

Your Recommended Grocery List

Proteins: You must have one at every meal. Try to buy organic when possible, especially red meat.

Beans (black, red, brown)	**Fish**	**Lean meats**	**Poultry**
	Cod	All-natural ham (nitrite free)	Chicken breast
Dairy*	Flounder	Beef	Ostrich
Cheese	Halibut	Buffalo	Turkey breast
Cottage cheese	Orange roughy	Lean pork	
Milk	Salmon (try canned)	Wild game	**Shellfish**
Natural yogurt	Tilapia		Crab (try canned crab instead of tuna)
Ricotta cheese	Tuna		
String cheese	High-quality whey protein		Lobster
Eggs, egg whites			Shrimp
			Tofu

*Pay attention to how you feel when you eat dairy. It can be an excellent protein source, but many people have an intolerance to it. If you feel bloated, lethargic, heavy, or gassy or have a stuffy or runny nose after you eat it, you should consider eliminating dairy from your diet.

Fruits and Vegetables: You must have one at every meal.

Alfalfa sprouts	Carrots	Green beans	Radicchio
Apples	Cauliflower	Jicama	Radishes
Artichokes	Celery	Kale	Raspberries
Arugula	Chard	Leafy greens	Red and green bell peppers
Asparagus	Chicory	Leeks	
Avocados	Chives	Lemons	Rhubarb
Bamboo shoots	Coconut	Lettuce	Sauerkraut
Bananas	Collard greens	Limes	Scallions
Beet greens	Cucumbers	Mushrooms	Snap peas
Blueberries	Edamame	Onions	Spinach
Bok choy	Eggplant	Oranges	Squash
Broccoli	Endive	Peaches	Strawberries
Brussels sprouts	Escarole	Peas	Tomatoes
Cabbage	Fennel	Pineapple	Water chestnuts
Cantaloupe	Grapefruit	Pumpkin	Zucchini

Starches

Cream of rice	Oats	Rice cakes (unflavored)	Wheat bran
Ezekiel bread	Potatoes	Sweet potatoes	Wheat-free breads made from millet, rice, rye, or spelt
Grits	Quinoa	Tortillas (corn, rice, spelt)	
Lentils	Rice (brown or wild)		

Fats: Don't worry about limiting fats on this plan. Enjoy with any meal!

Avocados	Flax oil, flaxseeds	Olive oil, olives	Raw cashews*
Butter (*not* margarine)	Herring	Pecans*	Raw walnuts*
	Macadamia nuts*	Pumpkin seeds	Sunflower seeds
Coconut, coconut oil	Natural peanut butter*	Raw almonds, almond butter*	

*Nuts also have protein and can be used as a protein source for snacks.

Once your kitchen is devoid of junk and stocked with healthy fuel, the following are your Base Phase Fit Female Nutrition Rules to live by. We went over these in detail in Chapter 8. Stick to the following rules 90 percent of the time.

10 Fit Female Nutrition Rules to Live By

1. Eat breakfast within 15 minutes of waking up, followed by a meal every three to four hours.

2. Eat a high-quality protein source at every meal and eat a mixture of different proteins.

3. Eat a fruit or vegetable at every meal and snack.

4. Eliminate all processed carbohydrates.

5. Use healthy fats and oils freely.

6. Eliminate caloric beverages and drink half your body weight in ounces of water every day.

7. Eat whole foods instead of bars and shakes whenever possible, except immediately after a workout.

8. Supplement with a multivitamin and omega-3 fish oil daily.

9. Always drink a workout shake either during your workout or within 10 minutes of finishing.

10. Keep a journal and stick to these rules 90 percent of the time. Plan to splurge no more than 10 percent of the time.

These rules are your nutrition rules for life. These next four weeks are your opportunity to really get them down. Understand how your body feels when you're following them and start to see your body make the breakthrough to become fit and fabulous.

The menus below are only examples to give you an idea of what following the above nutrition rules should look like. You may want to start with these menus and then begin to substitute a different protein for a given protein (refer to your grocery list) or a different piece of fruit for the type of fruit that's mentioned. Do not feel that you have to stick to these menus as a rigid plan, but instead use them as a guide. In fact, feel free to design your own menus based on the rules and grocery list.

Base Phase Sample Menus Following the Basic Rules

Workout Day

MEAL	FOOD	SUPPLEMENTS
1	1–2 eggs, $\frac{1}{2}$ cup–1 cup oatmeal, 1 banana	Multivitamin, 2–3 grams omega-3
2	POSTWORKOUT: 1 scoop whey protein powder mixed with water, $\frac{1}{2}$ cup milk, ice, mango, and strawberries	
3	Romaine lettuce with olive oil and vinegar, chicken breast, apple	
4	Brown rice cake with peanut butter, small apple	
5	Asparagus, brown rice, 1 serving turkey	
6	Natural yogurt (no sugar added) with walnuts and blueberries	Multivitamin, 2–3 grams omega-3

Nonworkout Day

MEAL	FOOD	SUPPLEMENTS
1	1–2 whole eggs plus egg whites (have as many whites as you want to fill you up) with spinach and mushrooms, wheat-free toast, $\frac{1}{2}$ avocado, orange slices	Multivitamin, 2–3 grams omega-3
2	Cottage cheese with walnuts and cinnamon, sliced apple	
3	1 serving turkey breast on wheat-free bread with lettuce and tomato, handful of baby carrots	
4	Ground turkey chili made with black beans, bell peppers, and onions (make a big batch of this and keep it in your fridge)	
5	Broccoli, sweet potato, 1 serving lean steak	
6	2 hard-boiled eggs, cantaloupe	Multivitamin, 2–3 grams omega-3

"DEFINE YOURSELF" PHASE: WEEKS FIVE THROUGH EIGHT

This is the next step if you have been "eating clean" following the basic Fit Female Nutrition Rules for four weeks and have developed some good habits. You should be feeling a difference in your body, your energy, and your overall health. Your metabolism should be starting to increase, and your clothes should be fitting differently. You should be turning into a fat-burning furnace and beginning to look like the fabulous fit woman that you are!

Your body is smart, though, and will adapt to your nutrition just as it adapts to your training program. If you've been eating the exact same thing every single day and your progress has started to slow down, it's time to make a change. However, if you're still seeing results, don't mess with success! I am all for doing the least you need to do in order to achieve the result you want.

"If it ain't broke, don't fix it" rule. If the basic Fit Female Nutrition Rules are working, your body is shedding fat weekly, your workouts are going great, and you have energy and are feeling good, don't change a thing. You want to do the least amount you need to do to get the results you want. Hopefully, you can stick to those rules right to the end, until you are fit and fabulous. *However,* if your progress has started to slow down, you're hitting a plateau, or you're ready to increase your results, you should pay attention to the following changes and put them in place immediately. Once you get to where you want to be, you should be able to go back to the original fit female rules and stick to them 80 to 90 percent of the time for the long term, giving yourself at least 10 percent freedom to splurge.

Fit Female Nutrition: "Define Yourself" Phase

Continue with all the rules from the first four weeks, including eating whole food sources of protein and carbohydrates every three to four hours, incorporating fruits and vegetables in every meal and snack, and drinking your water. These next four weeks, make the following changes to the plan to keep your body from adapting.

1. **Time your starches.** *Nutrient timing* is one of the latest buzzwords in nutrition, because nutrition experts have found powerful effects of eating certain types of foods at certain times, and those of us in the fitness industry are learning how to take advantage of this so we can help our clients turbocharge their workouts with this valuable information. Start to time your intake of starchy carbohydrates according to when they'll benefit your body the most. This means eat starchy carbohydrates only for breakfast and after workouts, when your body is most depleted and needs them most. They must still be from unprocessed sources (such as rice, oatmeal, potatoes, and sweet potatoes). Your body is completely depleted two times a day—at breakfast and after your workout—and you want to hike your blood sugar up to a stable level as soon as possible. First thing in the morning, you should have a starchy carbohydrate with protein, such as oatmeal with eggs. Also, after your workout you should have a shake containing protein and carbohydrates, and then about an hour to two hours after you have that shake, eat a meal with protein and a starchy carbohydrate (such as chicken with rice) to top off your glycogen stores. Glycogen is the storage form of carbohydrate in your muscles and gets used up

during a workout. Other than these two times, do not consume starchy carbohydrates. Instead, you should use only fruits and vegetables as your carbohydrate sources at other meals and snacks.

"There is no such thing as good or bad food, just good or bad times to eat certain foods."

—UNKNOWN

2. **Limit your fruits.** Keep fruits to no more than two servings a day for this phase only. I've noticed that some of my clients end up eating too much fruit. Although fruit is a very beneficial fit female food, it does have sugar in it, so you have to be careful not to overload on it. Limiting yourself to two servings a day during this phase will keep your body changing and still give you the benefits fruit has to offer.

A client of mine was following the Fit Female Nutrition Rules from Phase One and wasn't losing weight. She said, "I'm following it exactly, sticking to everything." I usually see people respond quickly when they adhere to these rules, so I started to ask questions and found out she was consuming five bananas a day. She loved bananas, and I hadn't told her she had to limit her banana intake, so she was having five a day. Limit your servings of fruit to two per day while you're trying to lose fat, and the rest of the day, eat vegetables at every meal.

3. **Follow the 90 percent rule.** Be honest with yourself: Have you really been following the Fit Female Nutrition Rules? Go back to the journal you've been keeping. (You have been keeping a journal, haven't you?) Give yourself a check mark if you followed the nutrition rules or an X if you missed a meal or did not keep to the rules. You must have 90 percent check marks to see results. Following these rules 90 percent of the time will put you well on your way to being fit and fabulous. This allows you 10 percent of the time to splurge. Enjoy your splurges! Don't feel bad about them. Just get back on track at your next meal. When you decide to go out and have a good time, relax and enjoy it. After a little while, you'll find that because you have been eating healthily, you'll feel better and won't have cravings for junk food. It won't be hard to keep your splurges to a minimum, but give yourself the freedom to indulge if you want to.

90 Percent Rule

As long as you are trying to change your body, you must stick to the Fit Female Nutrition Rules 90 percent of the time. This means . . .

✦ If you have five meals a day, seven days a week, you have 35 meals at which you can decide to either stick to the rules or splurge when you want to. To change your body, 90 percent of these meals need to conform to the above rules. This means 10 percent of the time you have room for missing a meal or eating something that doesn't exactly fit within the rules. With 35 meals, 10 percent means you get three to four of these meals to splurge with each week.

I asked one of my clients what she had for breakfast one morning, and she said, "Eggs and potatoes." Sounded like a good breakfast to me. As a coach, I've learned that the more questions I ask, the better, to get to the bottom of things. So I asked her what kind of potatoes, and she responded, "Tater Tots." Tater Tots are no longer potatoes; they are processed food. Just check the ingredients and you'll see that the second ingredient is hydrogenated fat, followed by a few more ingredients that you can't pronounce. Tater Tots are not on your grocery list.

IMPORTANT: Be honest with yourself. Eating french fries or Tater Tots counts as a splurge, even though they have potatoes in their ingredients. Don't justify foods you know you shouldn't. Also notice I said, if you miss a meal, it counts as one of your 10 percent splurges. Do not waste a splurge on missing a meal. You may as well eat something, rather than miss a meal. The way I see it, I would rather you eat the wrong thing than eat nothing at all, because at least it will keep your metabolism up and you won't end up in a state of total starvation. Remember, the state of total starvation is a very dangerous state to be in, because you'll start to rationalize a binge on something you don't even want.

Fit Female Splurge Grid

At this point you can simplify your journal by using what I call a splurge grid, like the one shown below. Go through each meal for the week and give yourself a check mark if you followed the rules and an X if you missed a meal or had a splurge. What percentage of check marks did you get? Ninety percent? This concept was first introduced to me by John Berardi, Ph.D., who calls it a compliance grid, and it's been a very useful tool when it comes to keeping track of how closely clients are following what I tell them to do. I find that most women, when they think they are doing everything right and they can't figure out why their bodies aren't changing, are usually between 60 percent and 70 percent compliant. Your body will not change unless you are following the rules 90 percent of the time. So, when you tell me you're following the rules "most of the time," I can guarantee if you check your splurge grid, you're probably at 70 percent—not acceptable.

You also *must* have a postworkout shake. Give yourself a check mark each time you do. If you work out and do not have a postworkout shake, it counts as an X.

X = Missed a meal or splurged

✓ = Followed the Fit Female Nutrition Rules

The goal is 90 percent ✓s to change your body. (Four Xs allowed per week.)

MEAL	MONDAY	TUESDAY	WEDNESDAY	THURSDAY	FRIDAY	SATURDAY	SUNDAY
1							
2							
3							
4							
5							
Postworkout shake							

"Define Yourself" Phase Sample Menus
Workout Day

MEAL	FOOD	SUPPLEMENTS
1	1 banana, 1–2 eggs, oatmeal	Multivitamin, 2–3 grams omega-3
2	POSTWORKOUT: 1 scoop whey protein powder mixed with water, ½ cup milk, ice, and pineapple	
3	1 serving chicken breast, brown rice pasta, marinara sauce, red bell pepper	
4	Ground turkey chili made with black beans, bell peppers, and onions (make a big batch of this and keep it in your fridge)	
5	Mixed vegetables, 1 serving mahi mahi	
6	Handful of almonds, celery	Multivitamin, 2–3 grams omega-3

Nonworkout Day

MEAL	FOOD	SUPPLEMENTS
1	Buffalo patty, spinach, potatoes in olive oil	Multivitamin, 2–3 grams omega-3
2	Natural yogurt (no sugar added) with blueberries and slivered almonds	
3	1 serving turkey breast, lettuce, bell pepper, olive oil, vinegar	
4	Celery with peanut butter	
5	Green beans in olive oil with garlic, grilled chicken breast	
6	Cottage cheese with walnuts and cinnamon, sliced apple	Multivitamin, 2–3 grams omega-3

"DIAL IT IN" PHASE: WEEKS 9 THROUGH 12

At this point, you are eight weeks into your fit female transformation. Your workouts are getting tougher and tougher. Your body is responding, and you're feeling really good about yourself and how you look. For the next four weeks, once again to keep your body from adapting, we will start to cycle your carbohydrates.

The "If it ain't broke, don't fix it" rule is still in effect.

Fit Female Nutrition: "Dial It In" Phase

1. **Eliminate dairy and nuts.** This means your grocery list no longer includes milk, cheese, cottage cheese, peanut butter, almond butter, or any kind of nuts. These are good sources of protein and fats, but the calories can add up. From now on, they count as a splurge. Once you get to where you simply want to maintain your fit female body, you can add them back in.

2. **Manipulate your carbs.** Eat lower-carbohydrate foods for three days and then have one day of higher carbohydrates.

Carbohydrates give you energy and help retain muscle (and muscle is a metabolism booster, so we want it), yet they can also stimulate fat storage. When you eat fewer carbs and replace those carbs with protein, the body ramps up fat-mobilizing enzymes and hormones, resulting in accelerated fat loss. However, a prolonged period of low carbs will leave your muscles weak and lacking in glycogen. Going too low carb for too long depletes your glycogen.

What does this look like?

Days 1 through 3: Take in protein, a vegetable, and a good fat at every meal. Postworkout, you should have a workout shake that includes fruit and whey protein. Do not consume any starchy carbohydrates for these three days and stick to only 2 servings of fruits.

Day 4: Add a starchy carbohydrate for breakfast, add one to the meal following your workout, and include one more starchy carb in your dinner. Along with these starchy carbohydrates, you should also add two more pieces of fruit on this day. This will not work as well if you don't eat higher carbohydrates on this day.

"Dial It In" Phase Sample Menus

Low-Carb Day: Follow for Three Days

MEAL	FOOD	SUPPLEMENTS
1	Turkey patty, 1–2 eggs, spinach, pineapple	Multivitamin, 2–3 grams omega-3
2	MEAL REPLACEMENT OR POSTWORKOUT: 1 scoop whey protein powder mixed with water, ice, and pineapple	
3	1 chicken breast, lettuce, red bell pepper, olive oil, vinegar	
4	Ground turkey chili made with black beans, bell peppers, and onions (make a big batch of this and keep it in your fridge)	
5	Mixed vegetables, 1 serving mahi mahi	
6	Celery, turkey breast	Multivitamin, 2–3 grams omega-3

High-Carb Day

MEAL	FOOD	SUPPLEMENTS
1	1–2 eggs plus egg whites (have as many whites as you want to fill you up), natural ham, spinach, and mushrooms wrapped in a large spelt tortilla; grapefruit	Multivitamin, 2–3 grams omega-3
2	MEAL REPLACEMENT OR POSTWORKOUT: 1 scoop whey protein powder mixed with water, ice, pineapple, and peach	
3	Turkey breast on wheat-free bread, lettuce, bell pepper, peach	
4	Tuna, cucumber	
5	Asparagus in olive oil with garlic, grilled chicken breast, baked potato	
6	Natural yogurt (no sugar added) with raspberries	Multivitamin, 2–3 grams omega-3

FINE-TUNE PHASE: WEEKS 13 THROUGH 16— BE THE BITCH!

These are the final weeks of your fit female transformation.

WARNING: I know it's tempting for some of you to jump straight to this phase and get as strict as you can because you already eat pretty healthily. I strongly recommend that you start with the Base Phase and really nail the basics and speed up your metabolism. Many of you who have been chronic dieters need to feed your bodies for four weeks and get your metabolisms revving before you jump into this final phase. The final phase won't work if you haven't taken the time to get the basics down and get your metabolism up. Got it?

It's time to really fine-tune everything, push yourself in the gym, not miss a workout, and shed the last couple of pounds of fat while you build a few more pounds of lean body mass to really get that metabolism revving, making it easy to maintain your new fit female figure!

The "If it ain't broke, don't fix it" rule is still in effect.

Fit Female Nutrition: Fine-Tune Phase

1. Increase your fish intake to at least twice a day. Adding more fish will promote speedier fat loss. Research from France showed that when people substituted six grams of fish oil for six grams of fat, keeping their total calories the same, they burned more fat and lost an average of two pounds of fat in the following three-week period. Fish is also an excellent source of lean protein. Boost your fish intake to boost your fat loss.

2. During this final phase, you may have to start looking at the number of calories you're consuming to really dial it in. As I mentioned earlier, until you have all the other Fit Female Nutrition Rules figured out, you do not need to worry about counting calories. Now that you've built habits of eating like a fit female, to shed the last few pounds of fat, you may need to count your calories. Bottom line is, if you're consuming more calories than your body is burning, you will not burn fat. Up

until now, we've been relying on the fact that your body is going to burn more and more calories because of the muscle you're building. Also, your nutrition is naturally going to be the number of calories you should be eating, because you are eating healthy foods. But sometimes it is necessary, once everything else is in place, to look at the numbers but only for a short period of time while you dial it in.

How Do You Figure Out Calories?

There are complicated equations and high-tech devices to try to figure out the number of calories you should eat, but for the purposes of this book, to turn you into a fit female and not a physiologist, we will KISS—keep it simple, sweetheart:

Your body weight × 9 = calorie intake
for 3 days in a row which will be your lower food intake days (Low Days)

Your body weight × 15 = calorie intake
for 1 day to give your body a boost and keep it from adapting to the low days (High Days)

That's it. Keep it simple, sweetheart. For example, for a 150-pound woman . . .

Low day = 1,350 calories

High day = 2,250 calories

An excellent source for figuring out how many calories different foods have for this final phase is the website calorieking.com.

The key is that your high day (higher calorie,

higher carb), definitely needs to be a *high* day. There has to be a significant difference between your low days (lower calorie, lower carb) and your high days so you can trick your body and keep it guessing. Don't think you're doing better if you eat less on your high day. You must eat enough to give your metabolism a spike and keep your body guessing. Stick with the carbohydrate manipulation you started in the previous phase and use your high-carb day as your higher-calorie day and the other three days as low days. Take the total calorie number for a high- or low-calorie day and divide it by six meals a day, and per meal, that's what you should eat, along with continuing to observe the Fit Female Nutrition Rules you've already been following. Your metabolism should be revving by now, and dialing it in these last few weeks by keeping an eye on your calories and eating more fish will help you whittle off those last few pounds of fat.

Fine-Tune Phase Sample Menus

Low Day (Low Calorie, Low Carb): Follow for Three Days out of Four

MEAL	FOOD	SUPPLEMENTS
1	10 egg whites (egg whites are only about 10 calories each, so you can eat a lot of them and fill up on your low-calorie day), 3 ounces ground turkey, spinach, grapefruit	Multivitamin, 2–3 grams omega-3
2	MEAL REPLACEMENT OR POSTWORKOUT: 2 scoops whey protein powder mixed with water, ice, pineapple, and peach	
3	Lettuce, red bell pepper, olive oil, vinegar, 4–6 ounces mahi mahi	
4	1 can tuna, ½ green apple	
5	Mixed vegetables, 4–6 ounces orange roughy	
6	Cucumber, 3 ounces turkey breast	Multivitamin, 2–3 grams omega-3

High Day (Higher Calorie, Higher Carb): Follow for One Day out of Four

MEAL	FOOD	SUPPLEMENTS
1	4 eggs, butter, spinach, and mushrooms wrapped in a spelt tortilla; sliced pineapple	Multivitamin, 2–3 grams omega-3
2	MEAL REPLACEMENT OR POSTWORKOUT: 2 scoops whey protein powder mixed with water, ice, pineapple, and peach; natural yogurt (no sugar added) with blueberries and almonds	
3	8–10 ounces turkey breast on wheat-free bread, lettuce, bell pepper	
4	Romaine lettuce, olive oil vinaigrette, 8–10 ounces mahi mahi	
5	Green beans in olive oil with garlic, 8–10 ounces grilled salmon, baked potato	
6	Celery, 6 ounces chicken breast	Multivitamin, 2–3 grams omega-3

Again, once you have attained your fit body, go back to following the basic Fit Female Nutrition Rules for the long term. Don't obsess about counting calories, but focus on fueling your body instead. Counting calories is a strategy for these last four weeks, *and only if you need it*. Remember, if it ain't broke, don't fix it! Do not make a change if you are making progress.

WHAT ABOUT WHEN YOU'RE ON VACATION?

What I've found is that you can get away with one week of eating whatever you want, and be able to shed anything you gained within a week when you get back. The reason is that in one week the weight you gain will be water. No matter what you eat and how little activity you do you most likely will not gain fat in only one week. Plus, now that you are living the lifestyle and feel amazing you probably will end up eating fairly healthy anyway because you'll want to keep feeling fabulous. This allows you to go on vacation and totally relax, which I believe is very important, to give yourself a break from the rules.

Some rules you can keep in mind to keep the damage to a minimum:

1. **Still eat breakfast when you wake up,** and eat every couple of hours to keep your blood sugar stable. Even if you're eating junk, this will help keep you from being in a fat-storing mode and ending up in a state of total starvation.

2. **Have a protein at each meal.** Even if you're having pancakes for breakfast, order an egg to go with them. Again, this is all about keeping your blood sugar stable.

Relaxing and eating what you want, having a drink if you want to, and enjoying yourself are absolutely allowed. Who wants to watch what you eat when you're on vacation? There's a saying, "It isn't what you eat between Christmas and New Year's that matters; it's what you eat between New Year's and Christmas." This also rings true for vacations. You can take a week off, because the rest of the year, you eat and work out like a fit female, and when you come home from vacation, you'll get right back into your fit female routine. Taking a break from it for a week can give you a renewed motivation to dive back into it when you return—not a bad thing! Plus, once you are living the lifestyle and feeling great, you'll find that your vacations won't be the bloated food and drink binge-fests they used to be. Your body will be used to running on a certain type of fuel, and that's what you'll crave most of the time, especially if you're keeping your blood sugar stable by following the above two tips. You will have discovered that gorging yourself on a plateful of pancakes drenched in syrup will make you feel lethargic, bloated, and sluggish, and you simply won't want them like you used to.

One of my clients came to the gym after being on vacation and said to me, "We went out to my favorite restaurant, and I ordered what I usually order. But it didn't taste as good at all, and I just didn't enjoy it. I wish I would have ordered fish. I think I would have enjoyed it more. You have changed me!"

KEEPING YOUR PIPES CLEAN

I promised you I would not leave a single stone unturned when it comes to becoming fit and fabulous. One topic we haven't touched on yet is poop. We talked about how your urine should be clear and how if it's not, you're not drinking enough water. However, we have not discussed your No. 2 and the importance of keeping your pipes clean. What goes in must come out, and we should definitely touch on the subject. Your poop tells a lot about what your body is using and not using, and how healthy you are inside and out. Remember, your appearance on the outside is a reflection of what's going on inside. If you are constipated, have the runs, or have undigested food particles in your stool, these are all signs of something not being quite right. Pay attention to your habits. Like I said, as a fit female, you will be totally in tune with everything about your body. A fit female has a bowel movement at least once a day, and it should be solid and light brown, and shaped somewhat like a banana.

What some of the common poop problems might mean:

Constipation: This can be common when you change your food habits. Many times it takes a day or two for your body to figure out what all this healthy stuff is and what to do with it if it is a drastic change for you. But if the constipation persists, you may need more fiber or more good fats in your diet. Make sure you're eating enough fruits and vegetables. Remember, you should be having one serving of fruits and vegetables with each meal. If you don't think that's the problem, then it could be that you're eating too little fat. Add in some flax oil or some extra nuts and see if that speeds up the situation. Do not let yourself go for days without having a bowel movement. This is toxic and extremely unhealthy for you.

Diarrhea: This means everything is moving quickly. Your metabolism is up, but you may not have enough bulk in your diet. Up your fruits and veggies and fiber and you should see added bulk in your stool. If diarrhea persists, be sure to see a doctor, as it could lead to dehydration or be indicative of a bigger problem.

Undigested food: I don't mean to sound like your mother, but be sure you're chewing everything completely so your body can digest it. Your digestion starts in your mouth with chewing. If you are gulping down food without chewing, your body won't be able to process it. If you're chewing your food thoroughly and still see undigested food when you go, you may need to take some digestive enzymes to help break down the foods you're eating, so your body can get the full benefit of all the good stuff you're putting in it.

If You Are Having Digestive Issues, Consider Adding a Fiber Supplement to Your Arsenal

You should aim to take in 25 to 35 grams of fiber per day. Fiber is very important to reduce cholesterol, decrease the risk of colon cancer, and improve digestion. In addition to eating plenty of fruits and vegetables, taking a fiber supplement may also be necessary to ensure that you're getting enough of the nutrient. Use one or two scoops of a high-quality fiber supplement in one of your meal replacement shakes or sprinkled in your food. This will keep things regular! As we mentioned earlier, you don't want to let yourself get stopped up, which can be toxic and is not optimal for your body.

EVERY BODY IS DIFFERENT WHEN IT COMES TO NUTRITION AND FUELING

As you are making your breakthrough to become a fit female, you will get in tune with your body and how it responds to different foods. Use all the information above to figure out what works best for your body. You may tolerate more carbohydrates or not be able to tolerate them at all. Or maybe dairy doesn't sit well with you. Experiment and get to know your body and what it needs. Everyone is different and will need to tweak and make the above recommendations their own. Stay in tune with your body and how it's responding, and adjust accordingly. If your progress indicators are not showing progress, then make a change.

Chapter 10

Fit Female Workout Manifesto

All this talk should have you ready to take action. At this point you should be focused, motivated, and ready to hit the gym to start building your best fit female body and gaining all the confidence and empowerment I keep talking about.

The programs in this book have not only been well thought out but have also been used over and over again with actual females in the gym who live in the real world and have produced results. I myself have done them, and hundreds of women in my gym have followed a program very similar to the one in this book. There's a definite purpose to every exercise, every repetition, and every set. The programs in this book are based on the very program templates we have used successfully with our clients at our gym. In fact, while writing this book, I am taking a group of six women through this exact program and turning them into fit females. In addition, the model you see doing the exercises in the photos also took 16 weeks to follow this exact program herself.

I always tell my clients there is a method behind the madness. Let's talk about some of the principles and philosophies that shape the workouts you're about to follow. It's important to understand the following concepts in order to truly become a fit female. You can apply the same concepts to create new routines or to vary these routines. As long as you understand the following basic principles and keep them as part of your training, you will have success in your quest to become a fit female.

PRINCIPLE #1: PRIORITIZING YOUR WORKOUTS

Remember back in Chapter 1 we discussed "not having time" as no longer being an excuse? The programs in this book are written with time management in mind, using the most effective tools to carve out your fit body in the least amount of time. Most women don't have hours and hours to spend exercising, so this is where we look at the hierarchy of fat-loss training to explain the choice of workouts in this book and how you should prioritize your workouts. This idea of a hierarchy of fat loss was coined by my husband, Alwyn Cosgrove. Most women have their priorities flipped when it comes to their workouts: They prioritize their aerobic workouts, and if they have time, they fit in strength training as a last priority. As we discussed in Chapter 3, women need to start prioritizing strength training instead and change their paradigms regarding exercise.

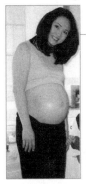

▲
Holly before

Holly whipped her post-pregnancy body into the best shape of her life losing 20 pounds of fat and 2 clothing sizes. ▶

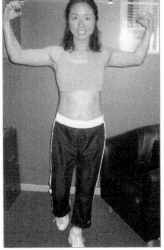

FIT FEMALE *Real Life Story*

After my second pregnancy, my body grew in ways unimaginable!

Initially, I sought the help of Rachel Cosgrove for vanity reasons, to get my body back in shape. However, I have stuck with her program now for the past eight years to promote the health of both my body and my mind. I consider working out regularly an investment in myself. I keep illness at bay and keep fit both physically and emotionally. I know I will age in good health and have the longevity in life that I seek as a mother of two. ✦

We have the following choices of exercise methods when it comes to burning fat and creating a fit body:

1. Metabolic Resistance Training, Also Known as Strength Training

What it achieves: Burns calories during the workout, maintains and builds lean muscle tissue, and boosts metabolism to the point of sizzling. You will burn more calories from now on because of the increase in your lean muscle tissue and therefore the increase in metabolism. This is good stuff.

What it does not achieve: Nothing! There is nothing strength training does not accomplish to get you closer to becoming fit and fabulous. Strength training offers the most benefits toward achieving a lean, fit body. And there is nothing you can't get from a strength workout.

As you can see, resistance training does everything you need it to do. Basically, you're using resistance training as the cornerstone of your workouts. Our goal is to work every muscle group hard, frequently, and with an intensity that creates a massive "metabolic disturbance" that leaves the metabolism elevated for several hours postworkout.

Metabolic disturbance: Remember in Chapter 1 we discussed that being in your comfort zone, doing what your body is already used to, means you'll stay the same? The goal of your workout is to put a demand on your body that it is not used to, taking yourself out of your comfort zone and creating a disturbance to your metabolism so your body will change. This disturbance includes breaking down muscle, up-regulating fat-burning enzymes and machinery, boosting hormones, and basically shaking up your system, resulting in burning a huge number of calories and giving your metabolism a boost to become sizzling. If you don't create enough of a disturbance, your metabolism won't increase as much.

What works best in our gym is full-body training in a circuit format with two to four noncompeting exercises (meaning upper-body then lower-body, so that whatever you just worked gets a rest) in a row and just enough rest to recover and begin the next exercise. Using a repetition range that's usually about 8 to 12 along with a load that is challenging creates the biggest metabolic disturbance and therefore the best results. We never do 25 to 30 repetitions during the strength-training workout, but instead save that for metabolic high-intensity intervals.

Using resistance training to gain or maintain your new muscle will make that muscle work harder and boost your metabolism, which will allow you to burn more calories. Remember, your goal is a sizzling metabolism. This is your No. 1 training priority in the fit female program. That's right, ladies, if you are going to miss a workout, do not skip your weight training. I'll say it again: It is your No. 1 priority!

2. High-Intensity Interval Training Cardio

What it achieves: This type of cardiovascular work burns calories during the workout and boosts metabolism to the point of sizzling.

What it does not achieve: High-intensity interval training provides all the benefits of strength training except that it does not actually put a high enough demand on your muscles to build lean muscle tissue.

The second key ingredient in achieving your fit chick body is high-intensity interval-training cardio workouts, which we also call metabolic workouts, because they are all about increasing your metabolism and becoming "metabolic," but not necessarily about building muscle. It all has to do with intensity—when you head out for a cardio workout, where is it on the intensity spectrum?

1. **Low intensity.** An easy pace. You could carry on a conversation, even sing a song, and could go forever at this pace. This is the most common form of cardio women do when they go for walks or jogs, but it's the least effective. See Chapter 3 again for why.

2. **Moderate intensity.** You're pushing yourself a little harder, but you could still hold this pace for a half hour to an hour or more. You could carry on a conversation, but in shorter sentences, and you couldn't sing a song. This will burn more calories than low intensity but is still not the most effective, because it won't increase your metabolism long term.

3. **High intensity.** This is where we want you for these cardio workouts: where you are increasing your heart rate to a point where you can't carry on a conversation and you can't hold the intensity for more than a minute or two. You are working hard, and you must recover before you can return to this intensity again. You could not do an hour of this type of workout.

High-intensity workouts burn the most calories. The downside is that they flat-out suck to do, because you have to push yourself out of your comfort zone! The upside is that these workouts eat up calories and increase your metabolism after the workout is over— the afterburn effect mentioned earlier, also known as EPOC (excess postexercise oxygen consumption). EPOC is defined scientifically as the "recovery of metabolic rate back to pre-exercise levels" and "can require several minutes for light exercise and several hours for hard intervals." What this means to you is that these are activities that keep you burning more calories after your exercise session. Bonus!

You can do metabolic interval-training workouts on a treadmill, a stairclimber, or any other piece of cardio equipment. However, I will tell you that that approach can get . . . *yawn* . . . boring, and I would rather you move your body in multiple planes of motion, challenging yourself with new movements. So the workouts in this book do not include any cardio machines, but instead use stimulating, calorie-burning body-weight circuits to really get your heart thumping! You should have plenty of metabolism-boosting exercises to choose from, but if you do decide to use a machine instead, pick one that challenges you, not the recliners (you know, the bikes that you practically lie down on).

3. Steady-State Cardio at an Easy or Moderate Intensity

What it achieves: This type of cardio burns calories during the workout, but that is it! You'll usually burn as many as 10 calories a minute if you're working pretty hard, so a whopping 300 calories in 30 minutes.

What it does not achieve: It does not increase EPOC, it does not build lean body tissue, and it will not increase your resting metabolic rate.

With tool #3, steady-state cardio work, we're just burning calories—we aren't working hard enough to increase EPOC significantly or to do anything beyond the session itself. But calories *do* count. Burning another 300-or-so calories per day *will* add up.

In my experience, I've found that many women have the hierarchy inverted. They do cardio and add weights later. Women typically make steady-state cardio their priority when it comes to exercise, but as you can see, it is the least effective in creating your fit body. It's the "icing on the cake" if you have extra time and energy. But who has extra time and energy? This is the least effective tool in your arsenal, as it doesn't burn much outside of the exercise session itself. Pick up those weights, ladies.

"A woman is like a tea bag. She only knows her strength when she is put in hot water."

—NANCY REAGAN

Time Management

So how does all this fit into your schedule? Let's talk time management and setting your priorities when it comes to your training. Start by figuring out how much time you can commit to your workouts, beginning with the end in mind and working backward.

If you have two to three hours per week, use only #1 above: metabolic resistance training.

This can be two or three one-hour training sessions or four 45-minute training sessions. I've had clients work out two hours a week, get their nutrition dialed in, and become fit and fabulous. Follow the programs in this book. The first two weeks, this is all you'll start with.

However, once you're getting three hours of total-body resistance training per week, you probably won't see an additional effect in terms of fat loss by doing more. At that point, recovery starts to become a concern, and intensity is impaired.

If you have four to six hours, use #1 and #2: weight training plus high-intensity interval cardio work.

This is what I've included in this book. At this point, when you're doing three resistance-training workouts a week, you can add in the metabolic workouts described. I'm looking to get you burning more calories and continuing to elevate your EPOC.

Interval training is like putting your savings in a high-return investment account. Low-intensity aerobics is like hiding the money under your mattress. Both will work, but the return you get is radically different.

If you have more than six hours available, add in #3: one or two aerobic workouts.

I think doing five to six hours a week is optimal for a fit female, and doing any more is not necessary unless you're really recovering well and just want to burn some extra calories. If you're not losing a lot of fat with six hours of training weekly, then I'd be taking a very close look at your diet. If everything is in place but you just want to ramp up fat loss some more (e.g., for a special event, such as a photo shoot or high school reunion), then you can add in some hard cardio—a long run or bike ride with your heart rate at 75 percent (or more) of maximum. But don't do more than an hour at a time unless you're training for an endurance event.

Why not do as much of this as possible, then? Well, the goal is to burn as many calories as you can without negatively affecting the intensity of your higher-priority activities. Just make sure this added cardio doesn't start to detract from your other workouts. Remember, your strength workouts are your priority, so if they suffer, you won't see the results you should. Oftentimes, less

is more, because the more you do, the less intensely you'll do it and the less effective it will be. So stick to less, but keep up the intensity.

PRINCIPLE #2: STARTING WITH A SOLID BASE

"Begin with the end in mind."

—STEVEN COVEY

Before getting specific, you must first build a solid base. At our gym we call it our corrective exercise phase, in which we address any existing weaknesses using basic strengthening exercises, including postural, core, and body-weight moves designed to increase range of motion and decrease the risk of injury. Think of it as if you are building a pyramid and you need a strong, solid base to build on top of. Starting with simple body-weight and postural exercises will set you up to be a fit female. Additionally, beginning your journey this way will allow you to safely perform every exercise down the road. The first program in this book has all the basic exercises you need to start off with a strong base. This is also the phase you'll come back to throughout your journey as a fit female. When you return to this phase a second time, you should be able to add load and increase the intensity of the workout while continuing to improve your base strength.

I see this all the time—a client joins our gym and sees other clients doing exercises that look really cool or more fun than what she's doing, because she's just performing "boring" corrective, body-weight postural exercises. I also see trainers get bored in the gym and start to give their clients more demanding moves before they're ready. But sticking to the basics for a longer period of time at the get-go will help you tremendously in the long run. The longer you stick to the basics, the better your foundation will be. And as a fit female, you should revisit the base phase frequently, but push yourself a little harder each time you do it.

Even if you've been training for a while, it's always a good idea to check in on the basics. Can you perform an overhead squat with good form? Can you lunge with good form and without pain? Can you row the same amount you can press?

"Success is a journey not a destination. The doing is usually more important than the outcome."

—ARTHUR ASHE

The first phase of the program in this book is about building a solid foundation. You should use body weight for most of the exercises the first time around, while you work on perfecting your form. The exercises in this first phase should help to correct some of the most common imbalances, to set you up with a solid foundation to build on. That's not to say this phase won't be hard—in fact, it's usually one of the toughest workouts, because you're targeting the muscles that aren't used to being worked.

PRINCIPLE #3: KEEPING THINGS IN BALANCE

The programs in this book are all balanced by movement patterns. They will not create an imbalance or an injury. In fact, they take into account the usual imbalances the average woman has when she joins our gym. Most women have similar behaviors including being on the phone, driving, being on the computer, holding children, wearing high heels, and sitting. These typical behaviors along with the way women are physically built have been taken in to account when I designed these programs to prevent injuries and help women to reach their potential. A woman should not do the same program as a man.

"I am very definitely a woman and I enjoy it."

—MARILYN MONROE

Some of the issues these female-specific programs address include the following:

✦ Most women are extremely quad dominant, meaning that they use their quadriceps (the muscles on the front of the thighs) much more than their butt and hamstrings. They usually have what's called gluteal amnesia, which I first learned about from strength coach Mike Boyle. Gluteal amnesia simply means they cannot fire their butt muscles when they need to—their brains have forgotten how to tell their butts to work. A common symptom of gluteal amnesia is the lack of a derriere. If you look at your body in profile in the mirror

SOME GOOD SELF-TESTS

✦ When you can perform 10 body-weight Bulgarian split squats, you're ready for weighted squats or deadlifts.

✦ When you can do 10 pushups, then you can move on to weighted bench presses.

Both of the above exercises, Bulgarian Split Squats and Pushups, are in the base program. When you come back to the base program a second time, you should be able to add weight or increase your range of motion on your Bulgarian split squats and progress with your pushups by doing them flat or on a decline (by putting your feet up on a bench) instead of on an incline, or by doing them on an unstable object. There are always ways to make every exercise more challenging. Start with the basics, then eventually progress.

and your butt is what we call a flat pancake ass, you may have a case of gluteal amnesia. This can lead to overuse knee injuries such as tendonitis, as well as ACL tears, which happen four to six times more often in women than in men. If you are missing a booty, this program will wake up your ass, literally! At our gym we are known for the butts we develop—I'm not kidding. I had a new client join, and on her second week she said, "I notice that all your clients who have been coming here for a while have the same butt. I want my butt to look like their butts. I want a Results Fitness butt!" This butt we're known for is strong, developed, and shapely. On this program, you will build a butt, and this is a good thing. We've been told we should call our gym Build-A-Butt.

✦ Many women also have the related problem of short hip flexors, usually due to too much sitting or too many hours on a spin bike. When the hip flexors are short, the hips are tilted forward and the posterior chain (butt and hamstrings) cannot work. Included in this program are exercises that actively lengthen the hip flexors, along with stretches to incorporate as a complement to the exercises.

✦ Most women also have forward head posture from all the hours they spend on the phone, in the car, and on the computer. Along with being the usual tension spot for us girls, where we hold all our stress, this quite often leads to shoulder or neck tension or injury.

✦ Most women have a love of shoes, and I'm not talking about super-supportive flats! I am talking about the lovely high heels we're so fond of wearing. What says confidence more than a woman sporting a pair of sexy high heels bringing attention to her defined legs? Yes, they make our legs look even better, but they come at a high price—dysfunction of the calves and tightness of the ankles, leading to issues at the knees and lower back. And if you wear them a lot, you may find that your body will adapt by placing more body fat on your rear end as a counterbalance, and your upper body will slump forward to compensate. I would never say that you can't wear them, after all they add to your fabulousness. I am saying that you should wear them only when you *must*. Regardless, we will be sure to undo some of this damage with the strength programs and stretching you'll be doing.

+ Most women have done too many crunches and not enough core stabilization exercises. They have poor core strength and lower-back stability. This is why you'll see a range of exercises for stabilizing the core and not a ton of crunches in these programs. Because females have wider hips, they usually have more of an anterior pelvic tilt (as we discussed above), meaning the top of their hips is tilted forward, creating tension in their lower back and many times causing back pain. A strong core can help correct this. In addition, a study in 2004 showed that core stability has an important role in decreasing lower-extremity injuries, which, as mentioned earlier, women are four to six times more at risk of having than men are. Core exercises need to be a staple in every woman's program and should be first priority, not last. Another research study of 23 women tested the order in which exercises should be performed and showed that whenever an exercise is done last in a training session, performance of that exercise will be negatively affected. Core exercises are extremely important and should be first in the program for a woman. Most women make the mistake of finishing their workout with their core work, never giving it priority.

+ Again, just us girls talking . . . right? Many women are settling for less sexual pleasure

these days, and are even heading toward urinary incontinence. Yikes! A recent study found that 25 percent of women (that's one in four!) between the ages of 20 and 39 already have bladder control problems, usually when they jump, cough, or laugh—how embarrassing! Many others have pelvic floor disorder known as prolapse, in which the organs in the pelvis, such as the uterus, fall down and protrude. Both are caused by having weak pelvic floor muscles. You can strengthen these muscles with strength training! This was shown in a research study that demonstrated a positive effect using pelvic floor muscle training in the treatment of prolapse. Many of the corrective and core exercises in the programs in this book will strengthen these muscles. Strengthening the pelvic floor can improve sexual function and enjoyment! Starting with the basics will give you a chance to learn how to engage your deep abdominal and pelvic floor muscles. Having a strong pelvic floor and core along with balanced posture is all part of being a fit female long term.

PRINCIPLE #4: HAVE A PLAN

"Failures don't plan to fail, they fail to plan."
—HARVEY MACKAY

The technical term in the training world for having a plan is *periodization. Periodization* means to have a plan of cycling the exercise demands to keep the body from adapting over a specific period of time to get to the desired result. The results we're looking for in this program are to turn you into a fit female. Many women don't know or don't care about the science of training. They may have heard about periodization, but they usually don't use it when designing their programs. A very common mistake I see many women make in their training is to do the same volume, the same weights, the same routine over and over again, without any plan to change it up and progress or change direction to a different volume and intensity. Periodization, or having a plan, has been scientifically proven to work and is something women need to include as part of a long-term, successful training program. Everything works, but nothing works forever.

Periodization consists of changing your training volume and intensity over periods of time to "peak" for a specific date or goal, such as a reunion or other big event. You can't continually push your body more and more, week after week, without giving it a back-off week to recover. If you continually push your body week after week, your body will eventually *make* you take a break by getting injured or getting sick. This will set your training back and can be avoided by using the science of periodization.

"It takes as much energy to wish as it does to plan."
— ELEANOR ROOSEVELT

The other component of periodization is being able to focus on improving one thing at a time. If you try to improve everything at once, nothing will improve. With a periodized program, you might spend four weeks focusing on building muscle in your upper body, and then the next four weeks building muscle in your butt and hamstrings while you maintain the muscle you built in your upper body. Then you might take four more weeks to really focus on burning fat and showing off all the muscle you've built. Try to do all this at one time and you won't accomplish half the results.

Shock your body—get out of your comfort zone! Change things up! Besides changing the loads, you must also change the stimulus to keep progressing while avoiding boredom and overtraining. I mentioned it earlier, but it bears repeating: You want to completely change your program every four to six weeks. You have to do what your body is not used to in order to get it to change. Your body adapts to the repetition range first, so this is the most important aspect to change frequently in your plan.

Our clients never get bored, and they never stop changing. Just when a client's body is getting used to a workout, we change it up. The fit female program changes every four weeks, so stick to the plan.

Does periodization have anything to do with your period? Well, periodization itself doesn't have anything to do with your period, but when it comes to your own plan, you will want to take your monthly reproductive cycle into account when scheduling your periodized workouts. We talked about this in Chapter 4,

Deciding What You Want and Why. The week before your period into the week of your period, you should try to be doing the lower-volume week of your four-week program, and the two weeks following your period, you should really ramp up and push yourself. Keep your menstrual cycle in mind with relation to where you are in your plan and adjust if necessary.

In this program, you'll have three weeks of building your volume followed by one week of recovery, when you cut your volume in half. The program will change every four weeks to keep your body from adapting to it. The program will also progress with each phase to include more challenging exercises and push you to new levels, in order to reach the final goal of becoming a fit female.

PRINCIPLE #5: USING "BANG FOR YOUR BUCK" EXERCISES

"Train movements, not muscles."

—VERN GAMBETTA

The fit female plan will use exercises that give you the most bang for your buck. By that, I mean exercises that give you the highest return for your training in the least amount of time, such as compound exercises that use a lot of different muscle groups, burn a ton of calories, and get more done at once. We will avoid using too many isolated exercises that take up time in your program without giving you as much

return. You should never train for longer than an hour at a time, so you have to fit everything into that hour. There's no reason for a female to waste time with biceps curls when her biceps will get plenty of work doing chinups and rows. Why would you want to isolate and just work on your biceps? They need to be in balance with the rest of your body anyway, so doing compound exercises will ensure that your biceps don't overpower the rest of your muscles, and you'll get more done at once. Some great "bang for your buck" exercises included in this program are squats, overhead squats, deadlifts, chin-ups, pushups, and bent-over rows.

PRINCIPLE #6: NO FIXED MACHINES

These programs do not use any stationary machines. Sitting on your butt on a fixed piece of equipment that moves in only one plane of motion, isolating one muscle group, is not part of my philosophy of what will turn you into a fit and fabulous female. Sitting on a machine will only further switch off your core and switch off your butt, and, as we just discussed, switching both of these *on* is one of the goals of this workout. Back to Principle #5—use "bang for your buck" exercises. We want to burn the most calories possible and work as many muscles as possible to build the body you want. Sitting on your butt on a machine will not accomplish this goal. A fit female does not do any seated chest presses, seated leg extensions, leg presses, leg

WEEK 1	WEEK 2	WEEK 3	WEEK 4	WEEK 5
Start a New Program	**Second Week on Program**	**Third Week on Program**	**Last Week on Program**	**(Week 1 on new program)**
1–2 sets only, lighter weights	Familiar with exercises, increase volume to 2–3 sets	Increase your loads	Personal record week	**Start a New Program**
Learn new exercises	Bump up your weights 10% on 2–3 exercises (not all of them)	Boost your intensity	Time to get everything out of the workout!	1–2 sets only, lighter weights
		Challenge yourself!	Going for maximum demand on your body to get it to change	Learn new exercises
		Bump up the weight again on 2–3 exercises (not all of them)	Use weights that you may not get every rep on every exercise. It is not necessarily the goal to miss reps, but push yourself with that intensity (keeping your form, of course)	**Notice:** Your intensity is lower, but is still a step up from 4 weeks ago
Intro Week	Base Phase Week	Overload Week	Shock Week	Intro Week

curls . . . or anything else that's done seated on a machine! The majority of the exercises in this program have you standing on two feet using multiple muscles, burning the most calories and getting the highest payoff for what you put in. The equipment includes dumbbells, barbells, a squat rack, cables, medicine balls, Swiss balls, kettlebells, and of course your body weight.

PRINCIPLE #7: UNDERSTANDING THE AFTERBURN EFFECT

The afterburn, or EPOC, is one of the primary goals of these fit female workouts: to create a metabolic effect that increases your metabolism so that you burn more calories and fat while you build muscle. Every workout needs to be at an intensity that will create a metabolic disturbance. The intensity of the workouts needs to be outside of your comfort zone to get you the results you're looking for.

What is the afterburn effect? An afterburn effect occurs when you have pushed your body during a workout at a high enough intensity to create a state in which you'll continue to burn calories at an accelerated rate for the next 24 to 48 hours. Usually after a workout that creates an afterburn effect, you may notice that you feel warm the rest of the day, because your body temperature remains elevated for a prolonged period of time. With every workout you do, your goal is to create this afterburn effect, stoking your metabolism to burn extra calories all day long.

PRINCIPLE #8: SAY NO TO AEROBICS

These programs do not include any steady-state, long, slow distance cardio. Zero! The programs call for only high-intensity strength-training workouts, along with two days of metabolic workouts (high-intensity interval workouts). Refer to Principle #1: Prioritizing Your Workouts if you have questions about this. You don't need to spend hours doing steady-state aerobics to become a fit female. Your body adapts to it too fast, and it becomes ineffective. Reread Chapter 3, Change Your Paradigms, Change Your Body, for a more in-depth explanation.

PRINCIPLE #9: STICK-WITH-IT-NESS

"We can do anything we want to if we stick to it long enough."

—HELEN KELLER

Stay the course. It's imperative that you consistently work toward your goal. It's always easy to start something, but not always as easy to finish. "Just do it!" as Nike says. If you want to reach your true potential, you have to be consistent day after day, week after week.

No matter how scientific your training program is or how much you know about fitness and training, the biggest key to seeing results from your training is simply showing up every day and getting it done. Sometimes people spend so much time reading websites, books, and magazines to get ideas for their training, they end up confused by all the different philosophies. When it comes down to it, the one principle they all have in common is that you need to get in the gym and train, day after day, week after week, and month after month. This book has a plan laid out for you—now get started and be consistent. Without consistency, none of this information will help you.

One of our clients had been training for about two years and was happy with the results but hadn't been really consistent with her diet and had missed a workout here and there. She had made progress but really wanted to see her body get to the next level. She would always bring in pictures from magazines showing girls she wanted to look like. She was already following a planned-out, individualized program, which included all the right exercises. She had built a solid base. Why wasn't she where she wanted to be? The answer was lack of consistency. So, she decided for the next 12 weeks she was going to be extremely consistent with both her diet and her training and see what happened. Guess what? She made so much progress, she was hooked and stayed consistent for another 12 weeks. We started to see her body transform before our eyes to look like every picture she had brought in from the magazines. It's amazing what a little consistency can do for you!

This also goes for your nutrition program. You can't start one plan and then decide you're doing a different plan on the weekend, and then Monday change your mind again. Decide on one plan and stick to it. Be consistent. Stick-with-it-ness is the key to seeing results.

PRINCIPLE #10: CREATE NEW DEMANDS EVERY WORKOUT

"To look like a fox, you have to sweat like a pig."

—Unknown (on a T-shirt I work out in)

What would happen if you did the same workouts over and over for a year? How long would it take before you'd stop progressing? This is why the amount of weight you use must increase to allow for continued physiological changes. After every workout, your body should recover and be stronger for the next workout. You should never lift the same loads twice. If you're recovering properly, you should be able to lift more weight every single workout, even if it's just an increase of ½ pound. Increase weight load for at least one to three exercises every single workout.

I don't want to hear "I don't want to get big and bulky" or "That's too much weight!" Hopefully, you are over this after reading Chapter 3 of this book and aren't worried about getting big and bulky. A good example of how big and bulky you'll become is a client of ours who just lost 70 pounds by progressively increasing her weights every week. Imagine that! She got smaller by get-

ting stronger every week. She went from incline-pressing the 15-pound dumbbells to lifting the 40-pound dumbbells and got smaller!

In fact, the only way to make any progress is to progressively increase your weights. If you're not getting stronger, you're not making progress. The only thing to be aware of about this is that you don't increase weight for every single exercise in one workout. Each increase will affect the exercises that follow in the workout. At most, increase weight for one to three exercises. And then, next time you do the program, pick a different one to three exercises to ratchet up. Push your body and challenge yourself to get better with every single workout.

"To learn, you have to be willing to push yourself."

—Brandi Chastain, professional soccer player

If you do what you've always done, you'll get what you already have! You have to learn to push your body beyond what it's already used to. Many women have a hard time doing this. There was a study which showed that women, when left on their own, would lift less weight than they were capable of. Learning to push beyond your comfort zone is a huge part of the success of this program. My goal is to get you comfortable with the fact that grinding out one last rep and grunting every once in a while is OK and may be necessary in order to create the body you want. Letting out an unintentional grunt is a happy accident of pure hard work, pushing your body beyond what it's used to. That's when your body will change.

I'm not saying women don't like to work hard. But it is rare to see a woman truly challenging herself in the gym, because most women have been conditioned not to. For some reason, women in the weight room pick up the rinky-dink dumbbells and do the exact opposite of what their bodies need to do to develop the look they want. Women have a higher pain tolerance than men (we all know this for sure; think about it—childbirth!); they just need to learn to apply it in the weight room. In our gym, you hear women grunting and groaning daily when they eke out that last rep of an exercise. They push their bodies beyond what they're used to during every workout. I forget that it's such an uncommon sight in a gym to see women lifting challenging weights, focused and training hard, because it is an everyday occurrence in our gym, and our clients have the bodies to show for it.

PRINCIPLE #11: AVOID CHANGING TOO MUCH, TOO OFTEN

As I just mentioned, you want to put new demands on your body every single workout, but you should stick to the same general program for four to six weeks. If you change the program too often, you won't see yourself progress. The new demands should come from increased loads and volumes. Stick to the same program long enough

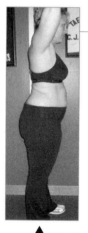

▲
Maria before

Maria as a fit female. She lost 70 pounds of fat and 6 sizes! ▶

FIT FEMALE *Real Life Story*

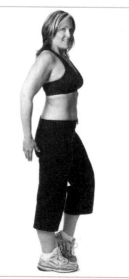

"I have worked to achieve the goals of being in great physical shape, losing weight, feeling good and looking good. After losing 70 pounds, and a total of 14% body fat I can say I am the happiest I have ever been." ✦

to achieve the benefits of that program, using the same exercises and numbers of repetitions for four to six weeks before changing.

Also, don't change everything at once. If you're starting a new strength-training program this week, then avoid overhauling your diet at the same time. Change one thing at a time or you won't know what is working. In this program, you'll notice that I start you off with three strength workouts per week. Two weeks later, I'll add in the interval-training workouts, instead of piling it all on at once. It's important to make things challenging but to continue progressing and seeing improvement each week with the same program over a four- to six-week period.

PRINCIPLE #12: SUPPORT AND ACCOUNTABILITY!

"Fit chicks of a feather, flock together!"

As women, we do much better when we have social support. We love our girlfriends and love to do things in groups. This is evident at any restaurant when one woman gets up to use the ladies' room and takes at least one girlfriend with her. So, what makes you think becoming a fit female should be done on your own? Reread Secret #10 in the Fit Female Credo, about having supportive people around you. Having support is your key to keeping your motivation and discipline to stick to your plan. How many times have you gone into the gym and talked

yourself out of doing that last set, or decided you didn't want to increase your weights that day, or just lacked the discipline to do the finisher you had originally planned to do at the end of your workout? This is where having a training partner or coach can really step up your results. Peer pressure can be a *good* thing.

This is one of our secrets at our gym—everyone works out in small groups. All of our training sessions are semiprivate, so our clients work out with at least one or two other people. I work with groups of up to 10 women at once and never work one-on-one with clients. Having a peer group along with a coach, our clients tend to work harder and feed off each other's energy. Nobody wants to let the group down.

If you have a hard time being disciplined, recruit a friend to join in on your quest. Find a friend who is not a crab and is supportive. A good fit female training partner will push you to do those last few reps or to stick to the program and avoid bailing out early.

"I never realized how much more weight I could lift and I love how strong I'm feeling. Typically my workouts were about how my physique would look, but with your plan, I get that and feel stronger. My posture is better and my legs tighter. My girlfriend and I are doing pullups (not by ourselves yet, but we're helping each other less and less). We also talk to each other constantly about our stress faucets and drains—it's like our therapy with each other!"—Megan, the model in the book

PRINCIPLE #13: KNOWING THE MEANING OF RECOVERY

"You don't get results from your actual workouts; you get results from recovering from your workouts."

—Unknown

You must have enough rest and recovery in order for your body to respond to the stimulus of training. Remember in the Fit Female Credo we talked about getting your R, R & R! Allow at least 24 hours between workouts and give yourself at least one day completely off every week to allow your body a full day of rest.

Usually three or four days a week of weight training is the most your body can handle and still recover. However, we have seen clients achieve amazing results in just two days a week. Just remember, more is not always better. You have to take into account your lifestyle and how much recovery you'll be getting. If you are a new mom and you're not sure you'll have a

YOUR BODY IS TELLING YOU SOMETHING

When you're feeling some tightness or soreness—this is like having a red light on your car dashboard and continuing to drive your car. Ignoring what your body is telling you is like ignoring that red light. Pretty soon another red light comes on or you feel something else, and eventually the car breaks down, just as your body will break down. If you fix the problem when it's just one red light, then it will never become a major issue. Becoming a fit female is all about listening to your body, getting in tune with it, and knowing when you need to back off. You need to pull over and fix the problem before you get back on the road.

chance to sleep through the night most nights of the week, two or three workouts a week will be plenty for your body to try to recover from. A hard workout won't do you any good if you don't recover from it. Listen to your body. If you feel that something is not quite right—a tight muscle or sore back—do not push through it. Your body will give you signals, and you have to listen before it turns into something major. Usually with a little stretching and foam rolling, you can fix the problem.

PRINCIPLE #14: KEEPING TRACK

We discussed progression in your workouts in Principle #10, and the only way you'll know for sure that you're managing this is if you keep track of what you've done. Go to the gym with a plan written down (you can photocopy the workouts from this book), and next to each exercise, write down what weight you lifted and how many reps of everything you did. Put the date down and any other notes about how you felt, whether the workout seemed easy or hard, and whether you had any issues come up. The next time you do the workout, you'll know exactly what you did last time and what you need to do to progress. Don't leave it to memory, because you won't remember how much weight you lifted or how many sets you did. Keep a journal and keep track of each workout and your progress.

FINALLY, LET'S GET STARTED!

Part 4

BUILDING YOUR FIT FEMALE BODY

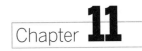

Chapter 11

The 16-Week Fit Female Workout Plan

All right, girls, time to build your fit and fabulous body! This training program is 16 weeks long and is broken into four phases:

Base Phase—Fit and Fabulous: This is the phase you'll come back to at any time throughout your training to keep your body looking gorgeous as ever. This is home base.

"Define Yourself" Phase: In this phase you'll see definition, tone, and shape happening in all the right places.

"Dial It In" Phase: Get ready to shed some major fat in this phase. Your body will change dramatically! Adding in a finisher at the end of each workout will give you an extra boost.

"Fine-tune" Phase: This is where you peak. Be the BITCH—be inspiring, totally confident and hot!

FIT FEMALES TURN HEADS

As you build confidence and begin to achieve the sexy look you want, you will draw the attention of the men in the weight room. Forgive them—they're not used to seeing a woman walk into the gym unintimidated, with a purpose, and looking confident while lifting weights.

You will probably turn their heads and get some attention (in a good way).

Stay focused on your workout, but enjoy the attention. After all, training to look and feel sexy is your goal, isn't it?

Do not get distracted. . . . unless, of course, you see Mr. Right!

Oh, and if you're already taken, you can still bask in the attention. Let it give you a boost of confidence and propel you through your workout!

You'll start with the base phase, and then you'll move through each remaining phase of the 16-week program with a different goal every four weeks. The first time you run through the 16-week program, do it in order and stick to each program for four weeks, starting with the base phase, and by the time you finish fine-tuning, you should be completely transformed and have made your own breakthrough.

Each phase contains two strength programs that you will alternate two to three times a week on nonconsecutive days. If your schedule is so jam-packed that you absolutely cannot fit in three workouts a week, you'll still change your body with two workouts a week. Just remember that two a week is the minimum number of workouts. Spare me the excuses.

Just get it done! By phase four, if your schedule allows, you'll work up to three strength workouts and two metabolic workouts, plus an optional cardio workout. Metabolic workouts consist of body-weight circuits designed to get your heart rate up and your metabolism revving so that you burn a ton of calories and create an afterburn effect.

NO TREADMILLS ALLOWED!

This program does not involve a single treadmill, not because I don't think you have access to one, but by choice. Walking or running in one direction, in one plane of motion, going nowhere in a steady state will not get you closer to your goal of being fit. Instead, the workouts I've designed will challenge you and your body to change, because they are completely different from what you've been doing. Get off the treadmill for 16 weeks and see what happens! I'm not saying you won't do cardio, but you will not set foot on a treadmill for the next 16 weeks. And you absolutely will not do any steady-state aerobics. If you decide to head out for a run or a bike ride, just be sure it's not taking away from your recovery and that it won't affect your training. During phase four you can add in a cardio session, but this should be short (under 30 minutes) and intense. It's best to do this outdoors and push the intensity.

These are all total-body workouts, so you'll

do them on nonconsecutive days, with no more than three strength workouts in a seven-day period. The workouts will change in every phase. Your body will be adapting constantly to the challenges you put it through, so it's crucial to change things up so you can stay one step ahead of it.

Part of my philosophy on how women should train is to train with a purpose. You will feel confident when you walk onto the weight-training floor if you know what you need to get done that day. This program gives you a purpose—you'll know exactly which exercises to do, how many repetitions and sets to complete, and how much rest you should take. (Sorry, girls, I didn't leave much time to chat with the boys between sets.) Stay focused and stick to your prescribed rest periods. Your purpose in the gym is to get your workout done so you can become fit and fabulous. You can flirt when you're finished, over postworkout shakes.

All right, let's get down to the nitty-gritty.

BASE PHASE— "FIT AND FABULOUS"

This is home base. You can come back to this phase at any time throughout the year. This phase has everything you need to get started, but it also has everything you need to maintain your fit body. The only catch is that you cannot repeat this phase twice in a row. You can come back to it as many times as you want throughout the year, but do not repeat it back-to-back. Also, each time you do it, you should be increasing the amount of weight you use and pushing yourself a little harder.

I know it can be intimidating to venture out of the cardio area and your usual aerobics classes and instead hit the weight-training floor, so we're going to start gradually. This first phase will use mostly body-weight exercises so that you can get started without heading straight for the squat rack. When you come back to this phase a second or third time, you can easily add weight to any of the exercises as you are getting stronger and your body is changing. As your confidence builds, we'll eventually get you to the point where you're pushing the guys out of the way to load up the bar for your deadlifts. As I mentioned earlier, you have to build a solid foundation before you can add a lot of weight anyway. You want to be able to lift your own body weight before you start adding additional weight with dumbbells and so on.

You'll also notice that I've prescribed a range of 10 to 12 repetitions in this first phase, meaning you'll start with 10 reps and then work your way up until you can do 12 reps of each exercise before you add more weight. This phase will improve your posture and set you up for success during the other phases. You'll begin the first two weeks with two or three strength workouts. During this phase, you can also perform a metabolic circuit one day a week in addition to your strength workouts, but don't start this until you've been following the strength-training plan for two weeks. Week three is when you can start the metabolic workouts if your schedule allows.

"DEFINE YOURSELF" PHASE

This four-week stint is all about adding definition. You'll lift weights that are challenging. The programs will bump up in intensity, and your reps will drop down to 8. The rest periods will be short, and the workouts will be tough. In this phase you'll really start to learn to dig deep and challenge yourself. Performing 8 reps will begin to build some muscle tone to give you the defined look you want, but this program will start to shed the fat quickly, too. You should really start to see your body changing during this phase. You'll also continue with a metabolic circuit one day a week.

"DIAL IT IN" PHASE

What do I mean by "dial it in"? I say "dial it in" when a client has been training consistently and eating healthily but is complacent and ready to bump up her workouts and clean up her diet enough to see her body get "dialed in." This will usually be followed by the fine-tuning stage, when the client will peak.

In phase three, you'll continue building muscle and working on your strength by starting the program with a heavy set of 6 reps that will require you to really push yourself. You should try to lift more weight every week on these first two exercises. As I mentioned earlier, you will *not* get big and bulky by lifting more weight. In fact, the more you demand from your muscles, the more metabolic disturbance you create, which causes a boost in your metabolism that allows your body to change. Don't hold back! After you perform the sets of 6, you'll move into three higher-rep, more metabolically demanding circuits. This phase will also include a metabolic finisher at the end of each workout and metabolic cardio circuits on opposite days from your strength training.

"FINE-TUNE" PHASE

This phase is actually about peaking. Your body fluctuates throughout the year because of life stresses, holidays, and whatever else is going on. We'll talk about this in Chapter 13, Maintaining Your New Body.

But for those times when you want to make sure you look and feel your absolute best, you'll use the fine-tune phase. You cannot be at your peak all year long. Don't get me wrong—you will feel good about yourself, being the fit female that you are, all year long, but it's not necessary to train as hard and diet

BY THE WAY . . .

Halloween is a perfect example of how women want to wear sexy clothes and feel good about their bodies. On Halloween, women have permission to show off their bodies, and man, do they! Feel good about yourself this Halloween and wear the sexy outfit you've always had your eye on but have never had the guts to pull off.

as hard if you're not peaking for some particular event.

What kind of event might you be peaking for? It could be a vacation, a reunion, or maybe a holiday party where you plan to wear your slinky black dress. Another big night to peak for is Halloween. For example, I have clients who dial it in (with the "dial it in" phase) about eight weeks out from Halloween, then begin to fine-tune four weeks out, in order to peak for Halloween so they can wear whatever sexy costumes they want and feel good about themselves.

This final phase is more advanced, beginning with a complex exercise. And because you're getting into great shape, we'll switch up your reps every week so your body doesn't get too used to anything. Your loads should change according to how many reps you're doing in a given week. This phase will also include a metabolic circuit on opposite days, and I've included one optional day of cardio. Your cardio workouts should be intense and should last 20 to 30 minutes, preferably outside; you might go biking, running, hiking, or

whatever you prefer. By the end of this phase, you will absolutely be at your best!

ALTERNATING WORKOUTS

Each phase has two different strength programs—workout A and workout B—which you'll alternate. The following is a guide to how your week should look, based on how much time you have available and what phase you're in. You can move these days around as long as you keep one day off between your workouts. If you prefer to work out on Sunday, Tuesday, and Friday instead, that would work, too. Use the following as a guideline. It's flexible—life happens. If you miss a workout, just get back on track the next day. *Do not beat yourself up!*

Remember Principle #1—observe the hierarchy of fat-loss training and prioritize your workouts with that in mind. Plan your week according to how much time you can commit and stick to it, even if it's only 2 hours a week.

Weeks 1–2

Three hours a week: This is what I recommend in the base phase. Make your strength training a priority for the first two to four weeks. After week four, if your schedule does not have room to squeeze any more in, you can continue this way for the duration of the 16 weeks and still get results.

Week 1

MONDAY	TUESDAY	WEDNESDAY	THURSDAY	FRIDAY	SATURDAY	SUNDAY
Strength workout A	Off Spend 15 minutes foam rolling and stretching.	Strength workout B	Off Spend 15 minutes foam rolling and stretching.	Strength workout A	Off Spend 15 minutes foam rolling and stretching.	Off

Week 2

MONDAY	TUESDAY	WEDNESDAY	THURSDAY	FRIDAY	SATURDAY	SUNDAY
Strength workout B	Off Spend 15 minutes foam rolling and stretching.	Strength workout A	Off Spend 15 minutes foam rolling and stretching.	Strength workout B	Off Spend 15 minutes foam rolling and stretching.	Off

Weeks 3–8

Four hours a week: As you are building your strength, incorporate a high-intensity interval-training metabolic workout if your schedule allows. If not, stick with three strength workouts. Four hours a week is what most of my clients do. This is a very doable schedule and will produce amazing results. You can stick with four hours a week for the duration of the program and become a fit female. The majority of our clients work out 4 days a week consistently.

MONDAY	TUESDAY	WEDNESDAY	THURSDAY	FRIDAY	SATURDAY	SUNDAY
Strength workout A	Off Spend 15 minutes foam rolling and stretching.	Strength workout B	Off Spend 15 minutes foam rolling and stretching.	Strength workout A	Metabolic circuit workout	Off
Strength workout B	Off Spend 15 minutes foam rolling and stretching.	Strength workout A	Off Spend 15 minutes foam rolling and stretching.	Strength workout B	Metabolic circuit workout	Off

Weeks 9–16

Up to six hours a week: Even if you have six hours available, slowly build up to this workout volume. Save it for the "dial it in" or fine-tune phase, when you have a base strength built up and are strong and ready to bump up your volume. The key with this much volume is to really keep an eye on your recovery and make sure you are getting your R, R, & R, as we discussed in the Fit Female Credo.

MONDAY	TUESDAY	WEDNESDAY	THURSDAY	FRIDAY	SATURDAY	SUNDAY
Strength workout A	Metabolic circuit workout	Strength workout B	Off Spend 15 minutes foam rolling and stretching.	Strength workout A	Metabolic circuit workout	Optional cardio workout (Do not start until you've been strength-training for eight to 12 weeks.)
MONDAY	TUESDAY	WEDNESDAY	THURSDAY	FRIDAY	SATURDAY	SUNDAY
Strength workout B	Metabolic circuit workout	Strength workout A	Off Spend 15 minutes foam rolling and stretching.	Strength workout B	Metabolic circuit workout	Optional cardio workout (Do not start until you've been strength training for eight to 12 weeks.)

If time is not an issue, this is what I recommend:

Base phase, weeks 1–4 (two or three sessions a week): Perform two or three strength workouts *only*.

"Define yourself" phase, weeks 5–8 (three or four sessions a week): Perform two or three strength workouts *plus* one metabolic interval workout.

"Dial it in" phase, weeks 9–12 (four or five sessions a week): Perform two or three strength workouts *plus* two metabolic workouts.

Fine-tune phase, weeks 13–16 (six sessions a week, which is the most you're allowed): Perform two or three strength workouts *plus* two metabolic workouts *plus* one optional cardio workout if you need it.

Once you've been through the entire 16-week program, you can go back and jump around to whichever phase suits you best at that point in your training, but push yourself harder than you did the first time. The one rule is that you cannot repeat one phase two times in a row. Each phase has a different number of reps per exercise. Your body adapts to the volume of reps first, and this is why it's so important that you switch to a different phase every four weeks. Otherwise, your body will get too used to the number of reps, and you'll stop seeing progress. For example, you cannot do the fine-tune phase over and over again; it won't work back-to-back.

WARMING IT UP

Before each strength workout, you'll perform a dynamic warmup to get your body ready for what's to come. Now, I know what you're thinking . . . "I'll just skip the warmup, launch into the workout, and get going." Do not do this! The warmup is just as important as the rest of the workout. In fact, it's *part* of the workout. You will not get everything out of the workout if you don't do the warmup. This warmup is different from your usual walk on the treadmill for 10 minutes. You'll probably find that you won't know where your warmup stopped and your workout started, because your heart rate will be elevated and you'll be sweating right into the workout. The goal of the warmup is to increase your body temperature, get your endorphins and adrenaline flowing to stimulate your nervous system, increase the blood flow to the muscles, and increase your range of motion and flexibility for the targeted exercises you're about to do. By the time you begin your first work set,

your body and mind will be ready to go.

Perform the following straight through without stopping, to get your body warmed up and ready to go before every workout. This part of the workout will stay the same through every phase and will take you 10 to 15 minutes to perform. It may look like a ton of exercises, but it won't take you long at all. As you get to know it, you'll churn through it quickly and be warmed up and ready to train hard! Every exercise listed is there for a reason, so do not skip an exercise. With this warmup, everything will get stretched out, switched on, given an increased range of motion, fired up, pumped with blood, and ready to go!

Warmup

> Squat to Stand—10
>
> Heel to Butt—10
>
> Jumping Jack—20
>
> Crossover Lunge—10
>
> Lateral Jump—10
>
> Inverted Hamstring—10
>
> Single-Leg Forward and Back Hop—10
>
> Lunge Walk with Rotation—10
>
> Single-Leg Lateral Hop—10
>
> Inchworm—10
>
> Lateral Lunge—10
>
> Bent-Over Y-T-W-I—5
>
> Bridge March—15
>
> Lateral Band Walk—20

Exercise Descriptions for Warmup

SQUAT TO STAND

START: Stand with you feet wide apart and your arms reaching overhead as high as you can.

MOVEMENT: Good morning, good afternoon, good day, body! You'll feel everything waking up doing this movement. Keeping both arms reaching overhead, bend at the hips to touch the floor between your feet, keeping your legs straight to stretch out your hamstrings (the back of your thighs). Keeping your hands on the floor, drop your hips down into a squat position. Staying in a full squat position, reach up with your right arm and then with your left arm, so that you're in a full squat position with both arms overhead. From here, stand up, return to the starting position, and repeat.

HEEL TO BUTT

START: Stand with your feet shoulder-width apart and your arms at your sides.

MOVEMENT: Bend your right knee, bringing your right heel to your right butt cheek, and grab your foot with your right hand. Balancing on your left foot, keep your right knee pointed down to the floor and feel a stretch in your right quadriceps and hip flexor. Alternate sides for a total of 10 on each side. Really take a second to stretch each time. Don't rush through it.

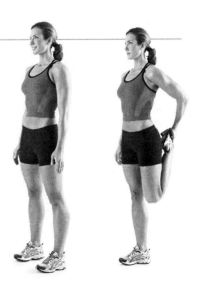

JUMPING JACK

START: Stand with your feet together and your arms at your sides.

MOVEMENT: Twenty jumping jacks will get you started! This is to get you moving and start the blood pumping without your having to think too much. Jump and land with your feet wide while you swing your arms up to form an X with your body. Each time you jump out, your heels should hit the ground. Jump back to the starting position as you drop your arms back down to your sides, and repeat. It's an old-fashioned jumping jack!

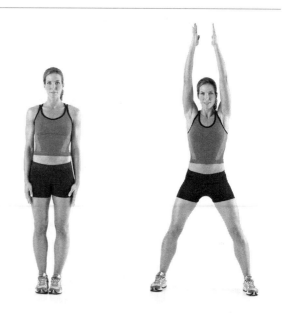

CROSSOVER LUNGE

START: Stand with your feet shoulder-width apart and your arms at your sides.

MOVEMENT: Cross your right foot over your left and step about two feet to the left of your left foot. Bend both knees, in a movement very similar to a curtsy. Keep your hips facing forward. You should feel a stretch across your right hip as you lunge. Return to the starting position and repeat on the other side.

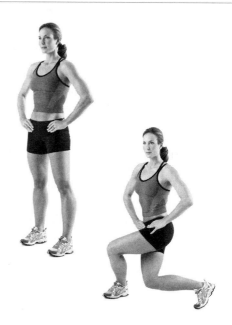

LATERAL JUMP

START: Stand with your feet together.

MOVEMENT: Imagine there's a line drawn on the floor to your right. With both feet, jump up and over the line and land on both feet. Pretend the floor is hot so that you land and jump right back over to the other side of the line. Keep your knees bent the entire time and explode back and forth. Wake up your nervous system!

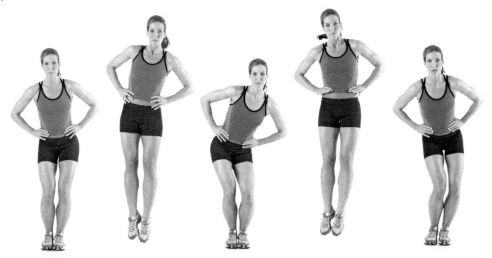

INVERTED HAMSTRING

START: Stand with your feet shoulder-width apart.

MOVEMENT: Step forward, putting your weight on your right leg. As if you were a teeter-totter, balance on your right leg and lift your left leg straight behind you while your torso bends forward to form a straight line from your head through your left leg. Keep your hips square. You should feel a stretch in your right hamstring. Bring your left leg down to the starting position and repeat on the other side.

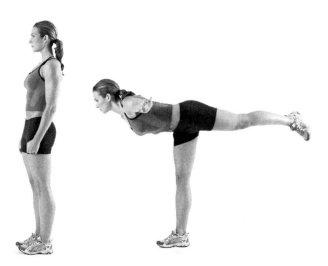

SINGLE-LEG FORWARD AND BACK HOP

START: Stand on your right leg.

MOVEMENT: Imagine there's a line drawn on the floor in front of you. Jump over the line with your right leg and land on your right foot. Then jump backward over the line to the starting position. Keep the jumps small and, again, pretend the floor is hot. Perform 10 on your right leg and 10 on your left leg. Again, you're waking up your nervous system!

LUNGE WALK WITH ROTATION

START: Stand with your feet shoulder-width apart and your arms at your sides.

MOVEMENT: Step forward with your right leg and lower yourself into a deep lunge. As you lunge, twist your torso over your right leg to increase the stretch in your left hip flexor. Return to the starting position and repeat with your left leg.

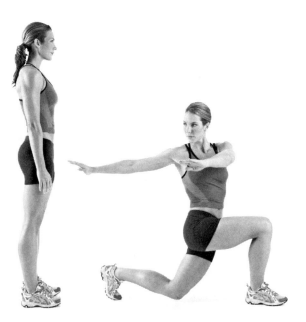

SINGLE-LEG LATERAL HOP

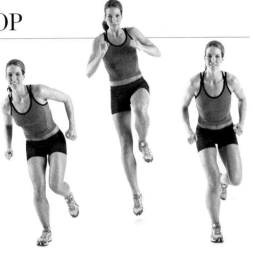

START: Stand on your right leg.

MOVEMENT: Imagine there's a line drawn on the floor to your right. Jump over the line with your right leg, land on your right foot, and then jump back over, still landing on the same foot. Keep the jumps small and, again, pretend the floor is hot. Perform 10 on your right leg, then 10 on your left leg (starting with the imaginary line at your left side).

INCHWORM

Now that you should be getting warm and breaking a sweat, this exercise will warm up your shoulders and core and get your entire chain ready to go.

START: Stand with your feet shoulder-width apart.

MOVEMENT: Bend at the hips and touch your hands to the floor as close to your feet as possible, feeling a stretch in your hamstrings. Walk your hands one at a time away from your feet and continue walking until you're in a pushup position. From there, continue walking your hands even farther, until you've walked out as far as you can while keeping your back flat. The goal is to eventually get your hands well past your head so you are completely stretched out. From here, walk your feet in toward your hands like an inchworm and repeat.

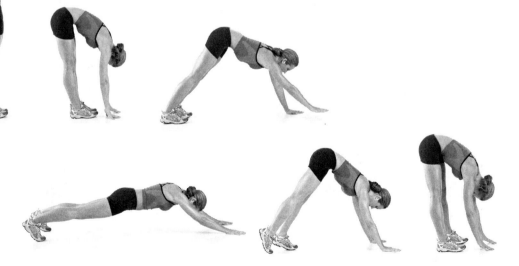

LATERAL LUNGE

START: Stand with your feet shoulder-width apart and your arms at your sides.

MOVEMENT: Step out with your right leg into a wide stance. Bend your right leg while keeping your left leg straight. Go as deep as you can go while keeping your right heel down. Try to get full range of motion, and then push off your right leg and return to the starting position. Repeat on the left.

BENT-OVER Y-T-W-I

Time to wake up your postural muscles!

START: Bend over at the hips with your knees slightly bent, your back flat, and your arms extended straight out so they form a Y with your torso.

MOVEMENT: Keeping your arms straight in the Y position, pull your shoulder blades toward each other to lift your arms slightly, then return them to the starting position. Repeat 5 times. Then take your arms straight out to the sides so your arms and torso form a T, with your thumbs rotated out to point to the ceiling. Perform the same shoulder-blade-contracting movement in this position 5 times. Then bend your arms at the elbow to form a W shape. Perform another 5 reps, pulling your shoulder blades toward each other and then releasing, to move your arms up and down. Then extend your arms straight past your head so your upper body forms an I shape, and again use your upper back to lift and lower your arms 5 times. By this time, your lower back and butt are probably also pretty warm from holding you in this position.

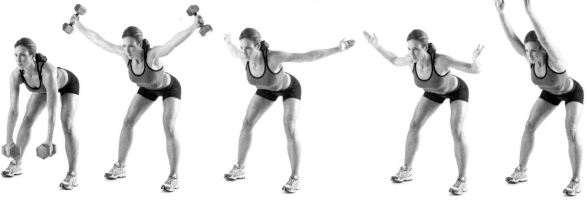

BRIDGE MARCH

START: Lie on your back with your knees bent and your feet flat on the floor. Lift your hips off the floor to form a straight line from your shoulders to your knees.

MOVEMENT: Maintaining that straight line, lift your right leg, then return it to the starting position and lift your left leg, and continue alternating. As you lift one leg, your opposite hip will want to drop, but keep your gluteal (butt) muscles contracted the entire time to hold your hips square. It's as if you're marching while keeping your hips extended. This is to wake up your glutes, as we discussed in Principle #3.

LATERAL BAND WALK

Last but not least, one final attempt to switch on your glutes and make sure you're warmed up and ready for the workout!

START: With a resistance band wrapped around your ankles, stand with your knees slightly bent and your feet shoulder-width apart, placing some tension on the band.

MOVEMENT: Keeping your knees slightly bent, step sideways with your right leg, increasing the tension on the band, and then step in with your left foot so your feet are the same distance apart as when you started. Continue walking to the right for 15 to 20 steps. Then repeat, walking to the left. Keep your torso as still as you can and just move from the hips. You should feel your hips burning and getting warmed up.

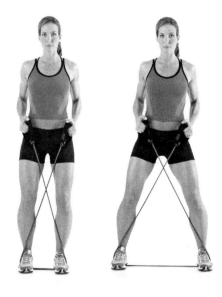

ALTERNATE YOUR SETS

Within the chart describing each program, for both the strength-training and the metabolic cardio workouts, you'll see that the name of each exercise starts with a number and a letter. Most of the exercises are in circuit style, meaning you'll perform more than one exercise in sequence, without resting in between. If you see the same number on two exercises (such as 1A and 1B), then those moves go together as a pair. You'll perform 1A followed by 1B, and then repeat 1A and 1B for a second set before you move on to the next circuit—2A and 2B. Sometimes you'll see a number without a letter following it, which means that exercise is done by itself. You'll also perform circuits of up to four exercises, such as 1A, 1B, 1C, and 1D. This means you'll do one set of each of these four before you start again with 1A and repeat.

A WORD ON REPETITIONS

The most common mistake I see women make when it comes to following a training program is that no matter how many repetitions the training program specifies, they grab the same dumbbells. For example, every time they do bench presses, they grab the 20-pound dumbbells, whether the plan says 8 reps or 15 reps or 20 reps. You see "bench press" and you think 20s. Most women lift too light for too many reps.

You must use a weight appropriate for the rep range you're working in. Your body will adapt to the number of repetitions first, so the program is designed with a specific number of reps in each phase, and that number changes in each phase for a reason. But if you don't lift enough weight for the number of reps specified, you won't put the demand on your body you need in order to get the results you're after.

Basically, you need to pick a weight that will challenge you for the number of reps specified. And whatever weight you use during the base phase for an exercise with 10 to 12 reps (stepups with body weight, for example), you need to grab a heavier weight in the "define yourself" phase, when you're doing 8 reps of the same exercise. (Grab a couple of 10- to 15-pound dumbbells for stepups in the second phase.) To become fit, you have to challenge your body every workout, so fewer reps calls for more weight.

Also, don't think you're doing me (or yourself) any favors because you knocked out an extra 5 reps above what I told you to do. If it says 8 reps, I want 8 reps with a weight that is challenging for 8 reps. So many women seem to think that more is better. The problem with this is that if the program says 8 reps and you do 12 reps, you'll have already been doing the rep range that's prescribed for the next phase, and your body will have already adapted to it. Stick to the program, ladies.

Moral of the story: Follow my instructions exactly regarding the number of repetitions of every exercise, and always use a weight that is challenging for that number of reps in each phase. Each week try to increase the weight and do the same number of repetitions.

TEMPO

The strength programs are all done at a moderate tempo, which means you're to move at a controlled speed. Take two seconds to lower the weight, hold for one second, and then take two seconds to lift the weight, hold for one second. Each rep should take you five to six seconds if you are doing it properly.

FINISHERS

Introduced in the "dial it in" phase: the finishers! Finishers are just that—moves to finish you off. They are demanding to your cardiovascular system, will give you an extra afterburn boost, and will finish you at the end of your workout. These are used in phase three but not in phase four, where instead we begin the workout with a complex (a sequence of moves done continuously without releasing or changing the weight).

Finisher A: Squat Thrust and Tuck Jump or Body-Weight Squat

This finisher involves squat thrusts in increments of three, performed as supersets (pairs of exercises) with either tuck jumps or body-weight squats in single increments.

For example:

3 squat thrusts

1 tuck jump or body-weight squat

6 squat thrusts

2 tuck jumps or body-weight squats

9 squat thrusts

3 tuck jumps or body-weight squats

12 squat thrusts

4 tuck jumps or body-weight squats, etc.

In weeks 9 through 12, you'll go up to 12 squat thrusts and then *back down* the ladder— so after 12 squat thrusts and 4 tuck jumps or body-weight squats, you'd do 9 squat thrusts and 3 tuck jumps or body-weight squats, etc.

Time the workout, and if you're up to it, rest twice as long as it took and repeat for another round.

Finisher B: Leg Matrix

Time yourself for:

20 body-weight squats to below parallel (meaning that at the bottom of the movement, your thighs are past the point where they're parallel to the floor)

20 alternating dynamic lunges with body weight (10 reps on each leg)

20 alternating lunge jumps

20 jump squats (thighs below parallel to the floor on the squats)

In weeks 9 and 10, during the "dial it in" phase, you'll perform one circuit of the above, time it, and rest twice as long as it took you to do it before repeating the circuit.

In weeks 11 and 12, you'll perform two circuits back-to-back before resting (you'll rest twice as long as it took you to do the circuits), then repeat for two more back-to-back circuits.

In the last phase you will not have finishers, but instead will start your workouts with complexes. You don't get an appetizer *and* dessert!

OPTIONAL CARDIO WORKOUTS IN FINE-TUNE PHASE, WEEKS 14–16

Once you've been strength-training for 12 weeks, have built up a base strength, have dialed yourself in, and are looking to fine-tune for an event, you can add in an optional cardio day if you feel you need it. During this cardio session, you should do no more than 30 minutes and keep it intense. Push yourself doing hill repeats running or on a bike, or find a tough hike to get your heart rate up. Your heart rate should reach at least 75 percent of maximum. Basically, you should not be able to carry on a conversation, sing a song, or do anything but grunt during this workout. Otherwise, if you go out for a walk or a nice, easy bike ride around the neighborhood, it's considered active recovery and is part of your active fit female lifestyle but does not count as a workout.

THE FIT FEMALE STRENGTH-TRAINING PROGRAM

Base Phase

Workout A

EXERCISE	SETS	REPS	TEMPO	REST
Warmup				
1A Bird Dog	2–3	10 on each side	1-3-1	30 seconds
1B Forward Ball Roll	2–3	10	Moderate	60 seconds
2A Stepup	2–3	10–12 with each leg	Moderate	30 seconds
2B Three-Point Dumbbell Row	2–3	10–12 with each arm	Moderate	60 seconds
3A Partial Co-contraction Lunge	2–3	10–12 with each leg	Moderate	30 seconds
3B Incline Pushup/Pushup	2–3	10–12	Moderate	60 seconds
4A Hip-Thigh Extension	2–3	10–12 on each side	Moderate	30 seconds
4B Bent-Over Reverse Fly	2–3	10–12	Moderate	60 seconds
Foam Roll and Stretch				

Workout B

EXERCISE	SETS	REPS	TEMPO	REST
Warmup				
1A Upper-Body Core Stability Russian Twist	2–3	10 on each side	Moderate	30 seconds
1B Prone Cobra	2–3	2–3	60–90 seconds	60 seconds
2A Overhead Squat	2–3	10–12	Moderate	30 seconds
2B Lateral Raise with External Rotation	2–3	10–12	Moderate	60 seconds
3A Single-Leg, Single-Arm Romanian Deadlift	2–3	10–12 on each side	Moderate	30 seconds
3B Split-Stance Cable Single-Arm Lat Pullover	2–3	10–12 with each arm	Moderate	60 seconds
4A Bulgarian Split Squat	2–3	10–12 with each leg	Moderate	30 seconds
4B Split-Stance Cable Row	2–3	10–12 with each arm	Moderate	60 seconds
Foam Roll and Stretch				

"Define Yourself" Phase

Workout A

EXERCISE	SETS	REPS	TEMPO	REST
Warmup				
1A Wood Chop	2–3	8 on each side	Moderate	60 seconds
1B Plank	2–3	60–90 seconds	Hold	60 seconds
2A Dumbbell Squat with Offset Load	2–3	8 on each side	Moderate	60 seconds
2B Dumbbell Alternating Overhead Press	2–3	8 with each arm	Moderate	60 seconds
3A Single-Leg Bent-Knee Deadlift	2–3	8 with each leg	Moderate	60 seconds
3B Chinup with Band	2–3	6–8	Moderate	60 seconds
4A Alternating Lateral Lunge	2–3	8 with each leg	Moderate	60 seconds
4B Two-Point Dumbbell Row	2–3	8 with each arm	Moderate	60 seconds
Foam Roll and Stretch				

Workout B

EXERCISE	SETS	REPS	TEMPO	REST
Warmup				
1A Reverse Wood Chop	2–3	8 on each side	Moderate	60 seconds
1B Prone Jackknife	2–3	8	Moderate	60 seconds
2A Stepup	2–3	8 with each leg	Moderate	60 seconds
2B T Pushup	2–3	4 each side	Moderate	60 seconds
3A Single-Leg Squat	2–3	8 with each leg	Moderate	60 seconds
3B Alternating Lateral Raise	2–3	8 with each arm	Moderate	60 seconds
4A Supinated Hip Extension with Leg Curl (SHELC)	2–3	8	Moderate	60 seconds
4B Inverted Row	2–3	8	Moderate	60 seconds
Foam Roll and Stretch				

"Dial It In" Phase

Workout A

EXERCISE	SETS	REPS	TEMPO	REST
Warmup				
1A Plank on Swiss Ball	2–3	60–90 seconds		60 seconds
1B Upper-Body Core Stability Russian Twist	2–3	10 on each side		60 seconds
2A Deadlift	2–3	6	Moderate	90 seconds
2B Military Press	2–3	6	Moderate	90 seconds
3A Forward and Back Stepover	2–3	15 with each leg	Moderate	60 seconds
3B Incline Dumbbell Bench Press	2–3	15	Moderate	60 seconds
3C Single-Leg SHELC	2–3	15 on each side	Moderate	60 seconds
3D One-Point Dumbbell Row	2–3	15 with each arm	Moderate	60 seconds
Finisher A: Squat Thrust and Tuck Jump or Bodyweight Squat				
Foam Roll and Stretch				

Workout B

EXERCISE	SETS	REPS	TEMPO	REST
Warmup				
1 Prone Cobra	2–3	60–90 seconds		60 seconds
2A Front Squat with Push Press	2–3	6	Moderate	90 seconds
2B Chinup	2–3	6	Moderate	90 seconds
3A Romanian Deadlift	2–3	15	Moderate	60 seconds
3B Dumbbell Push Press	2–3	15	Moderate	60 seconds
3C Barbell Split Squat	2–3	15 on each side	Moderate	60 seconds
3D Split-Stance Single-Arm Cable Row	2–3	15 with each arm	Moderate	60 seconds
Finisher B: Leg Matrix				
Foam Roll and Stretch				

"Fine-Tune" Phase

Workout A

EXERCISE	SETS	REPS	TEMPO	REST
Warmup				
1A Plank with Alternate Arm Reach	2	10 with each arm	Moderate	60 seconds
2A Complex: Deadlift, High Pull, Push Press, Reverse Lunge	4	8 of each move	Fast	90 seconds
3A Bulgarian Split Deadlift			Moderate	
Workouts 1 and 4	4	5 on each side		90 seconds
Workouts 2 and 5	2	15 on each side		30 seconds
Workouts 3 and 6	3	10 on each side		60 seconds
3B Single-Arm Dumbbell Chest Press on Swiss Ball			Moderate	
Workouts 1 and 4	4	5		90 seconds
Workouts 2 and 5	2	15		30 seconds
Workouts 3 and 6	3	10		60 seconds
3C Back Squat			Moderate	
Workouts 1 and 4	4	5		90 seconds
Workouts 2 and 5	2	15		30 seconds
Workouts 3 and 6	3	10		60 seconds
3D Chinup			Moderate	
Workouts 1 and 4	4	3–6		90 seconds
Workouts 2 and 5	2	10–12		30 seconds
Workouts 3 and 6	3	6–8		60 seconds
Foam Roll and Stretch				

Workout B

EXERCISE	SETS	REPS	TEMPO	REST
Warmup				
1A Swiss Ball Crunch	2	10–15		60 seconds
2A Complex: High Pull, Front Squat with a Push Press, Back Squat, Good Morning	4	8 of each move	Fast	90 seconds
3A Deadlift			Moderate	
Workouts 1 and 4	3	10		60 seconds
Workouts 2 and 5	4	5		90 seconds
Workouts 3 and 6	2	15		30 seconds
3B Dumbbell Rotational Overhead Press			Moderate	
Workouts 1 and 4	3	10		60 seconds
Workouts 2 and 5	4	5		
Workouts 3 and 6	2	15		30 seconds
3C Single-Leg Squat			Moderate	
Workouts 1 and 4	3	10		60 seconds
Workouts 2 and 5	4	5		90 seconds
Workouts 3 and 6	2	15		30 seconds
3D Bent-Over Row			Moderate	
Workouts 1 and 4	3	10		60 seconds
Workouts 2 and 5	4	5		90 seconds
Workouts 3 and 6	2	15		30 seconds
Foam Roll and Stretch				

REAL WOMEN HAVE CALLUSES!

Part of lifting weights and using iron is having calluses—rough spots on your hands. Your hands will develop calluses, especially as you are lifting heavier weights. You can wear gloves if you prefer. Otherwise, try using a pumice stone to buff off the toughened skin and keep your hands soft and feminine.

EXERCISE DESCRIPTIONS FOR THE WORKOUTS
Base Phase, Workout A

BIRD DOG

This is one of those exercises that you see someone doing and you think, "Big whoop! What does that do? Looks pretty easy!" And then you get down to do it and realize that you're dripping with sweat and shaking, and all you're doing is lifting your own leg and your own arm. I know, not very empowering, right? Well, the body it will give you is what is empowering!

START: Get down on your hands and knees with your spine in a neutral position (not rounded) and your stomach drawn in tight to recruit your abdominals and keep your torso stable during the exercise. You head should be in alignment with your spine.

MOVEMENT: Lift your right arm and your left leg straight out, extending your arm and lifting it so it's in line with your ear. Your leg should be straight out from your torso, so that you're squeezing your left butt cheek. Return to the starting position and repeat with your left arm and right leg. Alternate sides for the desired number of repetitions.

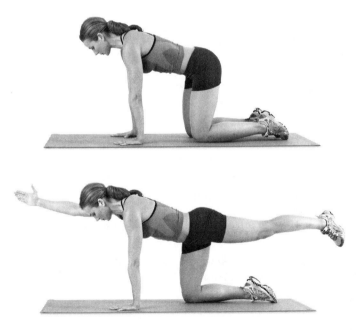

FORWARD BALL ROLL

Forget crunches! When it comes to building a six-pack, core stability is where it's at. This exercise will work your abs like you've never felt before. You will be sore, but you won't have to do 500 crunches. Sweet!

START: Kneel on the floor and place your forearms on a Swiss ball, drawing your abs in tight. Your upper arms should form 90-degree angles with your body, and your hips should be bent at a 90-degree angle.

MOVEMENT: Roll the ball forward by slowly extending your hips and arms, opening those 90-degree angles to eventually stretch out as far as you can while maintaining a neutral spine and keeping your abs tight. Be sure you're extending your hips and arms to equal degrees. Do not go beyond the point where you can maintain a stable back. If your back begins to arch, you've gone too far.

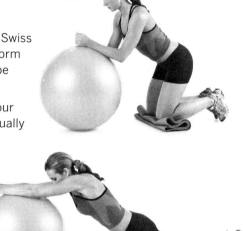

STEPUP

Forget the Butt Blaster machine! Chew on this—the Butt Blaster movement is the exact same movement as stepping onto a step, except that when stepping onto a step, you're lifting your entire body weight. If you can lift your body weight in that exercise, do you really think putting 10 pounds on the Butt Blaster machine and pumping it out for reps is going to do anything to change your body? No! For buns of steel, stick to stepups, and the taller the step, the more butt gets involved.

START: Stand facing a step or bench and place your right foot on the step.

MOVEMENT: Push through your right foot to lift your body up. Do not allow the trailing leg to touch the step. Lower yourself under control, pause briefly with your left foot on the floor, and repeat. Be sure to use only your right leg, and do not bounce or push off your left leg. Complete all reps on your right leg and then repeat on your left leg. Start on a low step and look to increase the height of the step as you gain strength. Then add load in the form of dumbbells.

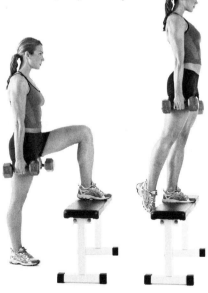

THREE-POINT DUMBBELL ROW

Ladies, we have to look good leaving the room, too! Tall posture and a strong, sexy back say "confidence." Nothing is sexier than being able to show off a toned, defined back wearing an open-backed shirt or dress. Performing a dumbbell row will give you a back you can feel confident leaving the room with.

START: Holding a dumbbell in your left hand, stand with a bench in front of you and bend over with your right hand supporting you on the bench. Your feet should be shoulder-width apart and directly under your hips, and your back should be flat, with your head, spine, and tailbone in a straight line. Your left arm should be hanging straight down.

MOVEMENT: Maintaining a neutral spine, raise the dumbbell toward you in a rowing motion by squeezing your shoulder blade. Lower the weight and repeat. Do not shrug your shoulder; the movement should all be from your back. After completing your reps with your left arm, change positions so that the bench is at your left side and repeat the move with your right arm.

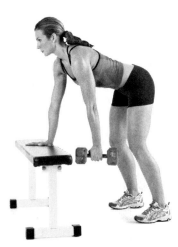 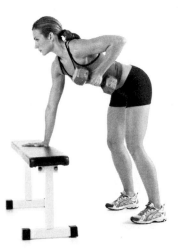

PARTIAL CO-CONTRACTION LUNGE

As I mentioned in Principle #3, most women are very quad dominant, meaning they use the muscles on the front of their thighs most and do not know how to fire their gluteal (butt) muscles, or glutes, along with their quadriceps. This exercise will teach your body to fire these muscles at the same time, which will train you to keep your knee tracking over your toe. This will decrease the potential for knee injuries while waking up your glutes. Your legs will burn doing this exercise! Push through, dig deep, and get all the reps you can!

START: Take a big step forward with your left leg and lower yourself into a lunge position by bending your left leg until your right knee touches the floor. Place your right hand on the teardrop-shaped muscle on the inside of your left knee, called the vastus medialis. Place your left hand on your left glute. Raise your right knee one inch off the floor and you'll feel the vastus medialis and the glute contract. This is the starting position.

MOVEMENT: Slowly raise yourself by extending both legs, all the time feeling for the tension in the vastus medialis and glute. The second you lose that tension (it probably won't take long), pause, then slowly return to the starting position (with your right knee an inch off the floor). Again, work only in the range where the muscles are contracting. Do not perform this exercise through any range where the vastus medialis and glute are not firing. Repeat for the prescribed number of reps or until total muscular failure, whichever comes first. Then repeat on the other side.

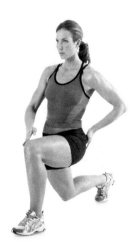
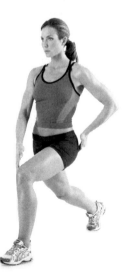

INCLINE PUSHUP/PUSHUP

No more "girl pushups"! From now on, you do real pushups. Incline pushups are a great way to eventually work up to doing pushups on the floor. As you get stronger, lower the incline until you're on the floor. Pushups not only work your upper body, including your shoulders and chest, but also are a great core stabilization exercise. The reason most women cannot do a pushup is that their core is not strong enough, not because they don't have the upper-body strength. Think about it—most women can do "girl pushups" on their knees; it's when we put them on their feet in a plank position using their core that they have trouble.

START: Assume a pushup position on an incline—that is, place your hands on a bar, bench, or wall to support your upper body, depending on how strong you are. If you're strong enough, begin in the standard pushup position, prone with your weight supported by your hands and your toes on the floor. Otherwise, the higher the incline on which you place your hands, the easier the pushup will be. Your spine should be in a straight line, with your head, upper back, and tailbone in alignment.

MOVEMENT: Bend at the elbows to lower yourself toward the floor, keeping your body in a straight line and your abdominals tight. Descend until your shoulders go just below your elbows, then return to the starting position, keeping your body in a straight line during the entire movement. If you cannot achieve the full range of motion without letting your back arch or sticking your hips out, then increase the incline.

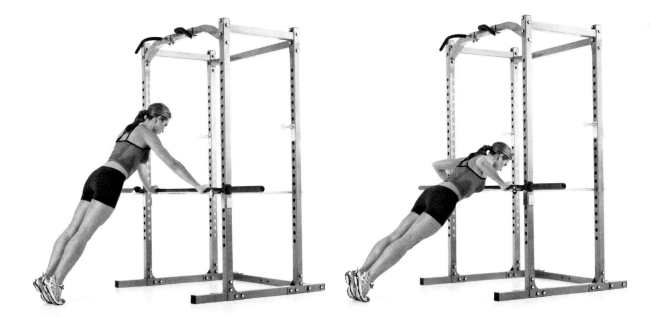

HIP-THIGH EXTENSION

If you don't focus on your butt, no one else will! No one wants a flat, flabby pancake ass. You want a strong, shapely, sexy derriere! You want a butt that men will not be able to keep their eyes off of. This exercise will help wake up the muscles in your rear and build a firm butt. Be sure to show it off with tight, fitted jeans that accentuate it just right. Nothing says "fit female" like a strong, sexy butt.

START: Lie on your back on the floor with your left leg bent 90 degrees, your left foot on the floor, and your right leg straight. Rest your arms on the floor, palms up, at 45-degree angles from your torso. Push off your left foot to lift your right leg, butt, and lower back one inch off the floor. This is the starting position.

MOVEMENT: Continue to lift until your entire body (except your left lower leg), from upper back to ankles, is in a straight line and your thighs are parallel to each other. The only parts of your body that should be in contact with the floor are your head, upper back, arms, and left foot. Lower yourself to one inch off the floor, pause, and repeat for the prescribed number of reps. Be sure to keep your hips in a straight line. Repeat on the other side. The extended leg can be bent, weighted with an ankle weight, or tucked to your chest as possible variations on this exercise.

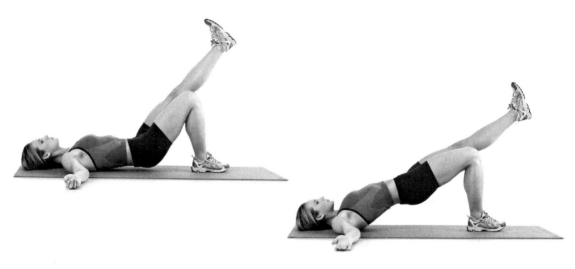

BENT-OVER REVERSE FLY

The taller your posture the more confident you look. Having excellent posture can actually make you appear 3-5 pounds lighter. This exercise was part of your warm up when you did the YTWI. If it was tough during the warmup then it is worth repeating with bodyweight only.

START: Bend over at the waist with your arms hanging straight down, lift your arms out to the sides squeezing your shoulder blades together by contracting the muscles in your back. Slowly lower to the start position and repeat for 10-12 repetitions. Add light dumbbells when you are able to perform 10-12 repetitions without using your traps, which are the muscles you use when you lift or shrug your shoulders. Your head and back should stay in a neutral position and your core should be tight. Avoid rounding your back as you start to get tired.

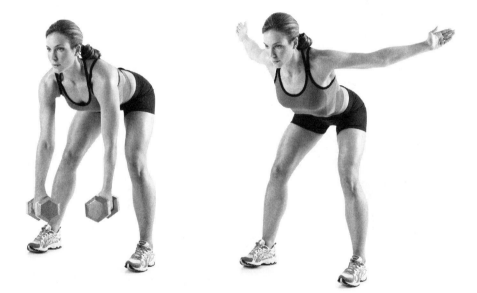

Base Phase, Workout B

UPPER-BODY CORE STABILITY RUSSIAN TWIST

Many women have poor core and lower-back stability as a result of a lack of proper core training. Learning to stabilize your core while lifting or moving a weight puts a demand on your entire core, which teaches you how to stabilize properly. This will keep your back strong and give you the lean, defined midsection you want.

START: Sit on the floor with your legs bent 90 degrees and your upper body leaning back slightly. Hold a small weight in your hands, extended out in front of you. To increase the difficulty, lift your feet off the floor.

MOVEMENT: Keeping your torso completely still, rotate the weight from side to side. To make the exercise more difficult, increase the range of motion, the speed, or the amount of weight you're using.

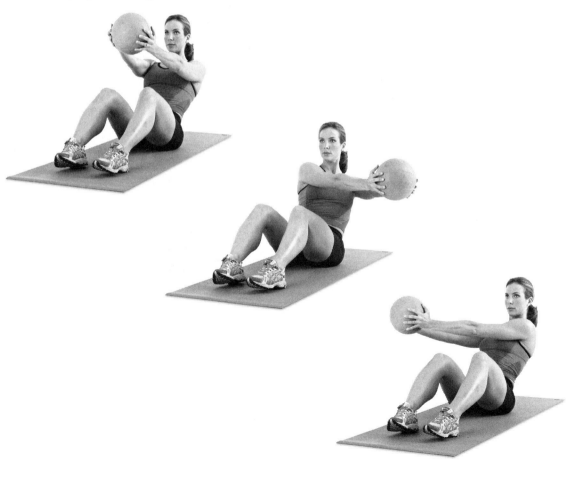

PRONE COBRA

Nothing says confidence like great posture. Standing up straight with good posture can take an instant five pounds off your appearance. This exercise will strengthen all your postural muscles, teaching you to stand up straight and look like the confident fit female that you are.

START: Lie face down on a mat or carpeted floor and rest your arms at your sides, with your palms down.

MOVEMENT: Contract the muscles in your butt and lower back so that your upper torso and legs come off the floor. At the same time, rotate your arms outward so that your thumbs end up pointed toward the ceiling. Keep a neutral neck alignment. Hold this position for 60 to 90 seconds. If you cannot hold for the recommended time, hold for multiple repetitions of five to 10 seconds. To make the exercise more difficult, you can hold dumbbells in your hands or perform the move while balancing on a Swiss ball.

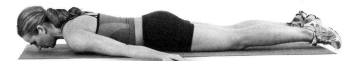

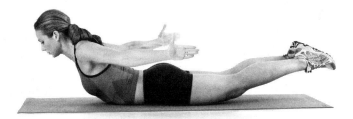

OVERHEAD SQUAT

Bet you never thought of doing squats to get a six-pack. By placing a weight overhead, you force your core to switch on to stabilize you. Not only that, but your shoulders (especially your rotator cuff muscles) have to work to stabilize the bar. Plus, this exercise will work your entire chain, meaning every muscle from head to toe will be engaged. This allows you to figure out the tight or weak parts of the chain, as they will show up as limiting factors in this exercise.

START: Set a bar in a squat rack above your head height. Until your strength increases, use a 10- to 20-pound bar or even a wooden dowel. You probably will not lift more than a standard barbell for this exercise. Progress slowly, starting with a wooden dowel to a light bar to a standard barbell. Grasp the bar with a wide overhand grip and lift the bar overhead by extending your arms straight up while bracing your abdominals. Your arms should be in line with your ears.

MOVEMENT: From this position, with the bar overhead, bend at the knees and hips and lower yourself into a full squat. Keep the bar in the overhead position with your arms locked up straight for the entire movement. Return to the standing position. As you squat, maintain a tall posture; don't let your back round, and keep your knees tracking over your toes. Don't let your knees collapse in toward one another. If you're having trouble performing a full-range-of-motion squat with your arms overhead, you are probably tight somewhere, most likely your ankles or your hips. Add a board under your heels to make the exercise easier. As your body becomes more mobile, you eventually want to be able to perform this exercise without a heel support. Repeat for the prescribed number of reps.

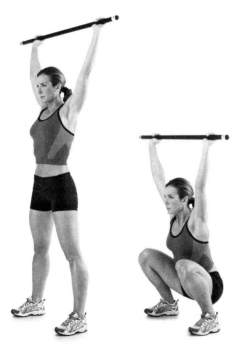

HOW LOW CAN YOU GO?

Before grabbing a bar, first do the overhead squat with your body weight only, arms overhead. How low can you go? You should be squatting with as full a range of motion as you can while keeping your heels down and arms overhead. If you need to put a board or two plates under your heels to increase your range of motion, you can. Once you figure out your range—how low you can go—then stay with it and do not decrease your range of motion when you add a bar overhead. Only use a weight with which you can keep the same full range of motion. And as you become more flexible, lose the heel lifts if you needed them.

LATERAL RAISE WITH EXTERNAL ROTATION

Nothing is less attractive than that small vertical roll of fat between your armpit and your chest. You know, that fold of fat that sticks out when you wear a tank top or hangs out of the side of your bra—yuck! I have heard it called "armpit fat" or "twinkies," and recently a client called it "bacon," because she said it is always the first to burn when she's in the sun in her bathing suit. Regardless of what you call it, nobody wants it! Building the muscles in your shoulders, chest, and arms will tone up this area so you can wear tank tops without worrying about the overhang. This is also an excellent exercise to strengthen your rotator cuffs and shoulder joints while improving your posture. Always a good thing!

START: Stand with your feet shoulder-width apart, with a dumbbell in each hand and your elbows bent 90 degrees (forearms pointing forward).

MOVEMENT: Maintaining the bend in your elbows, lift your arms out to the sides, keeping your wrists in line with your elbows. At this point, it looks like a lateral raise position with your arms bent. From here, pretend your elbows are sitting on a table and rotate your arms from the shoulder joints until your hands are directly above your elbows. Reverse the movement, still keeping your elbows stationary, then return to the starting position.

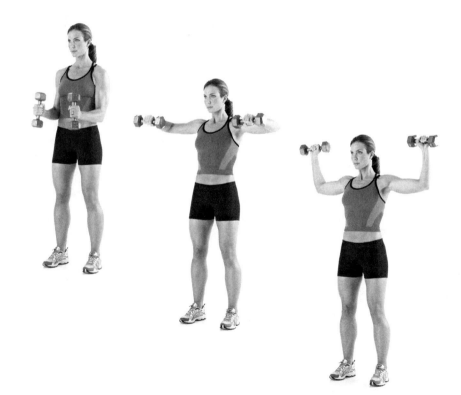

SINGLE-LEG, SINGLE-ARM ROMANIAN DEADLIFT

You have to train what you don't see in the mirror, too, ladies. This exercise hits it all: your entire posterior chain, or basically everything behind you—your upper back, lower back, butt, hamstrings, right down the chain! Feel confident turning your back.

START: Stand on your right leg with your left arm reaching out toward the ground in front of you. As you get stronger, you can hold a dumbbell. Stand with a neutral spine, which means do not let your back round.

MOVEMENT: Bending at the hip, reach for the floor with your left arm while pushing your hips back to stretch your hamstrings. Go as low as you can while maintaining a neutral spine, and then contract and return to the starting position. Repeat on your left leg, reaching with your right hand. Add a dumbbell as you get stronger.

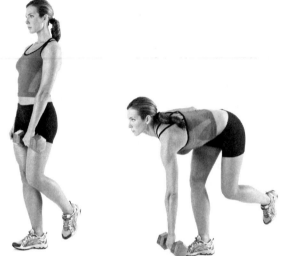

Use a kettlebell! If you have access to kettlebells, they work very well for this exercise because they are easy to actually set the weight on the floor each repetition. This forces you to really engage your glutes to lift the weight off the floor.

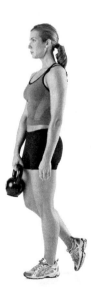

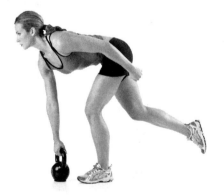

SPLIT-STANCE CABLE SINGLE-ARM LAT PULLOVER

You know when someone (hopefully a hottie) comes up behind you and wraps his arms around you (hopefully not only in your dreams) without warning and you are dying because you think he may have felt the fold of back fat before you got a chance to stand up straight and suck it in? This exercise works the muscle that runs from the back of your armpit to your lower back and wraps right around to the sides. Tightening this area will give you confidence to be caught without notice more often! Bring on the hotties!

START: Stand facing a pulley with a handle overhead. Your feet should be in a split stance with your right foot in front, your knees should be slightly bent, and of course your abdominals should be engaged (as if I were about to punch you in the stomach). Reach for the handle with your left arm.

MOVEMENT: The movement is all from the shoulder, not from the elbow. Tighten your abdominals to keep your core stable and pull the weight down as you keep your arm straight—move only from the shoulder—until the weight comes in contact with your left hip. Pause, then slowly resist as you let the weight pull your arm back up to the starting position. Keep your back naturally arched and your core very still and contracted as you perform the exercise. Also, remember to keep your shoulders down; don't shrug. Complete the set with your left arm, then switch legs and hands and repeat on the other side.

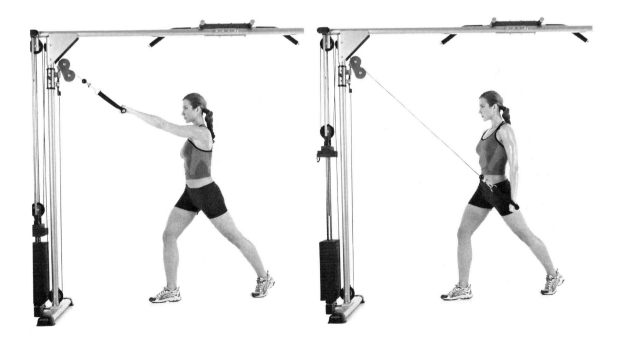

BULGARIAN SPLIT SQUAT

This is one of the most hated but most effective exercises in my gym. I usually tell my clients, "Hate me now, but love me later, when you're looking hot in your bikini on the beach!" A little visualization during this exercise might help get you through it. Think about the toned body you'll flaunt after you crank these out. This works the entire supporting leg while giving the other leg an excellent stretch. Nothing to it but to do it, ladies!

START: Stand with a bench behind you. Place your left foot on the bench and your right foot about two to three feet in front of the bench. You'll be in a modified lunge position with your torso upright.

MOVEMENT: With the bulk of your body weight on your right leg, bend your right knee until your right thigh is below parallel to the floor and your left knee is grazing the floor. Keep your weight on your right leg. Do not sit back and put weight on the left leg; that is cheating. Pause in the lowered position, then return to a fully upright stance. Complete the desired number of reps, then switch legs and repeat.

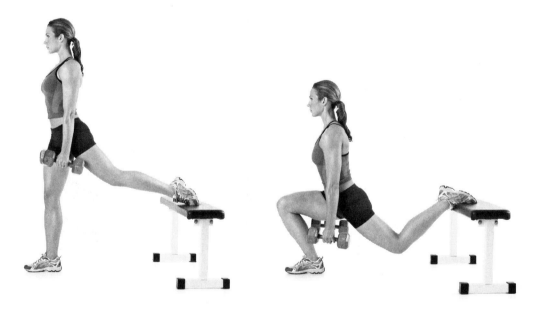

SPLIT-STANCE CABLE ROW

Most women spend far too much time with their posture rounded forward, whether they're talking on the phone, sitting at the computer, driving, lifting groceries or kids, cooking . . . I could go on and on. In any case, this creates an imbalance, which shows up as poor posture or eventually could create a shoulder injury or neck problem. Carrying more in the boob department will also pull your posture forward. I've also seen women whose breasts developed at a young age and were self-conscious of them, so they rounded their shoulders for so many years that this posture became deeply engrained in their bodies. All of the rowing exercises are designed to undo this forward, rounded posture and create tall, confident, empowered posture. Standing instead of sitting turns the move into a whole-body exercise that works your core and your legs to stabilize your body.

START: Stand facing a high cable pulley with handles attached, with your legs in a split stance, one foot in front of the other. Grasp the handles and position your body so your arms are extended straight in front of you and the weight is lifted just off the stack.

MOVEMENT: Using your back muscles, squeeze your shoulder blades together to pull the cable toward your body in a rowing motion. Keep your elbows in close to your body and keep your shoulders down. Pull the cable in as far as you can while maintaining your form. Pause, then slowly return the handles to the starting position by extending your arms as you resist the load.

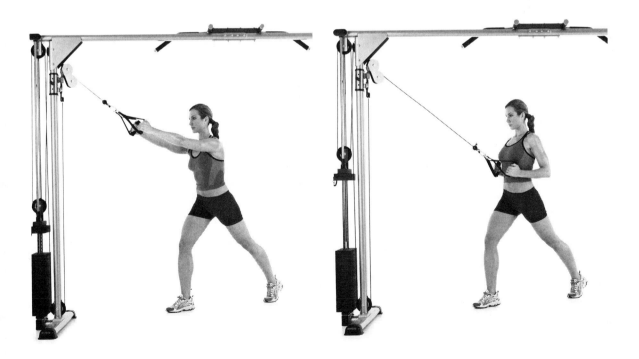

"Define Yourself" Phase, Workout A

WOOD CHOP

Most exercise programs neglect the transverse plane or movement rotating your body in one direction and then another. Working your body in the transverse plane is especially beneficial. When doing exercises like this, you are working your entire chain, using a lot of different muscles that are burning a ton of calories and getting your metabolism cranking. During this exercise you might want to think about that ex-boyfriend you can't wait to run into with your new hot body; the chopping motion might be more effective when you're thinking about someone you may want to get back at. Chop away!

START: Stand with a high pulley at your side and hold onto the handle with both hands and straight arms pointing up at a diagonal, ready to chop.

MOVEMENT: Keeping your arms straight, pull the handle across your body and down at a diagonal until your hands are on the side of the opposite hip. Keep your eyes on your hands as you do the movement. Return to the starting position under control and repeat to complete the set before switching positions to perform the move in the other direction.

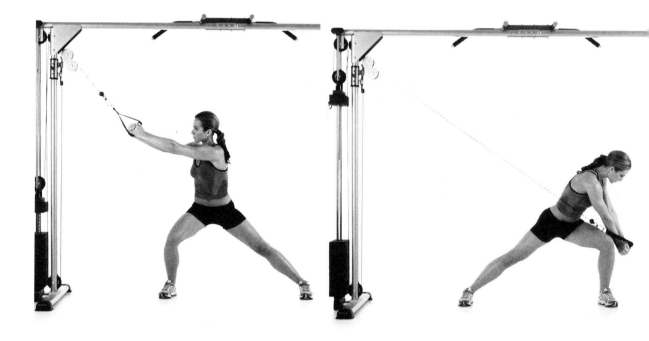

PLANK

This is another core stabilization exercise. Many women have a very weak pelvic floor, which can lead to trouble down the road, including pelvic floor dysfunction and bladder control problems. Doing core stability exercises will strengthen your pelvic floor and abdominal wall, reducing your risk of having these issues. And, perhaps most important, having a strong pelvic floor will increase your sexual pleasure!

START: Get down on the floor with your full weight supported on your forearms and toes, with your back in a straight line and your abdominals drawn in tight, keeping you stable.

MOVEMENT: There's no movement. This is a static exercise in which you hold this position without letting your back arch as you keep your abdominals tight.

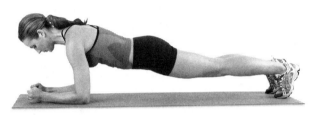

DUMBBELL SQUAT WITH OFFSET LOAD

Offset loads, or carrying something on one side of your body, are a part of life. We very rarely lift and carry something with two hands. Usually we lift a bag of groceries and carry it on our hip as we open a door, or carry a kid on one side, or lug around our purses that weigh about 20 pounds. It's important to train using movements we will do in our real lives. This is one of those movements.

START: Stand upright with your feet shoulder-width apart and hold a weight in your right hand, hanging straight down. Just standing there, you'll feel the left side of your body contract to keep you standing upright.

MOVEMENT: Keeping your body upright, resisting the weight pulling in one direction, lower yourself into a squat position by bending at the knees and hips through a full range of motion, until your hips are level with or below your knees. As you squat, be sure to maintain a tall posture; do not let your back round. And keep your knees tracking over your toes; don't let your knees collapse inward.

DUMBBELL ALTERNATING OVERHEAD PRESS

Gorgeous, defined shoulders and arms are a necessity for being a fit female. While performing these exercises, think about how you'll be able to show off your toned arms in a tank top. You are also switching on your abdominals every time a weight goes over your head, so not only will your shoulders get defined, but your abs will see some of that action, too!

START: Stand with your feet shoulder-width apart and a dumbbell in each hand, elbows bent so the weights are at each shoulder. Keep your chest tall and your abs engaged.

MOVEMENT: Push one arm at a time straight up overhead, then lower it. As you press the weight up, do not lean your body one way or the other. Instead, keep your torso perfectly still. Alternate arms for each repetition.

SINGLE-LEG BENT-KNEE DEADLIFT

This is a very important exercise for getting your glutes to fire to keep your knees from collapsing inward, which can create knee problems down the road. More women than men have anterior cruciate ligament (ACL) tears, and doing exercises like this will help reduce your risk. There is nothing sexy about ACL surgery.

START: Stand on your left leg. You can start with bodyweight only and then progress to holding two dumbbells for this exercise.

MOVEMENT: Bend at the left knee and hip, lowering your hips as you reach forward to touch the floor in front of you with your hands or dumbbells. Maintain a neutral spine, keeping your core tight. If you cannot bend all the way to the floor without rounding your back, go as low as you can while keeping your form. Start with light weights and work on your range of motion first.

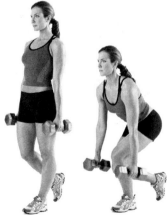

CHINUP WITH BAND

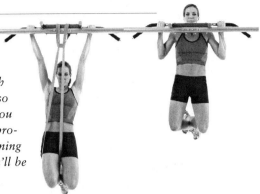

Women can do chinups—we just need to work at it. Chinups are an excellent exercise, and, surprisingly, if you've never done them before, you'll probably complain that you're sore all over, especially in your abdominals, which will be engaged along with everything else to pull your body up. The reason I love chinups so much is that they're a great example of how much strength you have compared with your weight. As you follow these workout programs and the nutrition advice, you will be losing fat and gaining muscle. Chinups will get easier and easier to do, because you'll be stronger and you'll weigh less!

START: If you're a beginner, 6 to 8 unassisted chinups might not be doable yet, so you can use a band for assistance. Hang from a chinup bar with a band looped around the bar and around one knee. Your hands should be facing you, and your arms should be fully extended.

MOVEMENT: Pull yourself up to the bar until your chin is over the bar, then return to the starting position. Think about bringing your elbows to your sides, which will ensure that you're using your back to pull yourself up. The band should act as support to help lift you up. The thicker the band, the easier it will be for you to pull up your body weight. Do not swing your legs or kick to cheat yourself up. As you get stronger, use a smaller and smaller band, until eventually you can ditch the band and do chinups on your own.

ALTERNATING LATERAL LUNGE

I'd better not catch any of you on one of those stupid inner-thigh machines again! They don't work. In case you haven't figured it out and are still using one, spreading your legs for the world to see, the machine will not work your inner thighs the way an exercise like this will. So get up, get on your feet, and start lateral lunging to tone up those inner thighs.

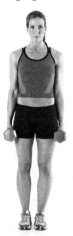

START: Stand with your feet together.

MOVEMENT: Step out to the right and bend that leg, lowering your hips while keeping most of your weight on your right leg. Push off that leg and return to the start position. Repeat on the opposite side.

TWO-POINT DUMBBELL ROW

This is a progression from the three-point dumbbell row you did in the base phase. Taking your hand off the bench will require you to use your back and hamstrings more to hold yourself in the bent-over row position. As you get stronger, it's important to slowly increase the difficulty of your exercises to keep your body changing in response to new demands. This will keep that back looking better and better, and you'll feel just as confident and empowered leaving the room as you do walking in.

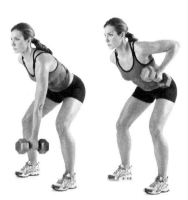

START: Bend over at the hips, holding one dumbbell straight down with one arm. Your back should be flat, with your spine in a straight line.

MOVEMENT: Squeeze your shoulder blades together to row the dumbbell up to your side, then return to the starting position.

"Define Yourself" Phase, Workout B

REVERSE WOOD CHOP

This is just the opposite of the wood chop we did on day one. This time you'll be chopping wood from the bottom of the motion to the top, once again working in that transverse plane that is so often neglected.

START: Lower a cable pulley handle to the bottom and, with straight arms, grab the handle with both hands. Your abdominals should be tight and your knees slightly bent.

MOVEMENT: Keeping your arms straight, pull the weight across your body at a diagonal, pulling from low to high. Keep your eyes on your hands as you do the movement. Return to the starting position under control and repeat.

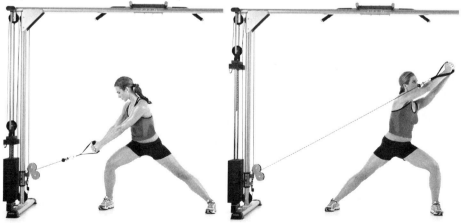

PRONE JACKKNIFE

Here's another way to work your abs without using plain old situps. Muffin top no more! A flat stomach and toned abs are supersexy. When doing these exercises, focus on how good you'll feel being able to wear low-cut jeans and a tight-fitting shirt, and maybe even letting your belly button peek out, showing off your flat stomach. Once again, by working to stabilize your core, your upper body and legs are also getting a workout.

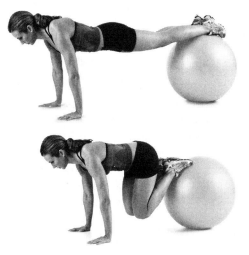

START: Begin in a pushup position with your arms straight and your feet on a Swiss ball. Your hips should be down, and your head, upper back, and butt should all be in a straight line.

MOVEMENT: Keeping your hips down and your torso completely stable, bend your legs to tuck the ball in underneath you, and then straighten your legs back out. Looking at you from the shoulders to the hips, it should look as if you're not moving; you're moving only your legs in and out. Do not let your hips come up.

STEPUP

Forget the Butt Blaster machine! The Butt Blaster incorporates the exact same movement as stepping onto a step. The only difference between the two is when stepping onto a step, you're lifting your entire body weight. If you can lift your body weight in that exercise, do you really think putting 10 pounds on the Butt Blaster machine and pumping it out for reps is going to do anything to change your body? No! For buns of steel, stick to stepups, and the taller the step, the more butt gets involved.

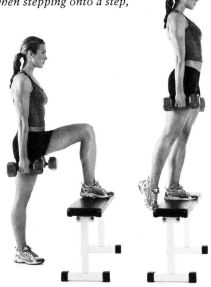

START: Stand facing a step or bench and place your right foot on the step.

MOVEMENT: Push through your right foot to lift your body up. Do not allow the trailing leg to touch the step. Lower yourself under control, pause briefly with your left foot on the floor, and repeat. Be sure to use only your right leg, and do not bounce or push off your left leg. Complete all reps on your right leg and then repeat on your left leg. Start on a low step and look to increase the height of the step as you gain strength. Then add load in the form of dumbbells.

T PUSHUP

I love this exercise, because it takes a great move—the pushup—and makes it even better! As I said earlier about pushups, they are a terrific core stabilization exercise, and this variation takes that core stabilization up another notch. This is an amazing exercise to work the core, shoulders, arms, and chest. (If you aren't ready for pushups on the floor yet, you can still do these on an incline with no dumbbells.)

START: Assume a standard pushup position.

MOVEMENT: Perform a pushup, then transfer all your weight to one hand as you rotate your body to reach up and behind you with the opposite hand. Keep both feet on the floor. Your arms should be in a straight line so that your body forms a T shape. Alternate sides. Once this becomes easy, lift both your arm and the foot on the same side off the floor after each pushup, so you make an X shape with your arms and legs. Holding hexagon-shaped dumbbells in your hands can also increase the intensity.

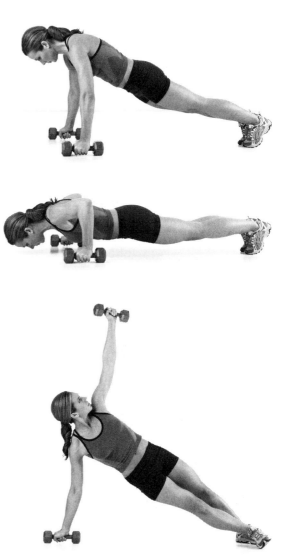

SINGLE-LEG SQUAT

This is one of the toughest lower-body exercises, and it's excellent for women. The goal is to eventually be able to do a full-range-of-motion squat standing on one leg. This takes a lot of strength and will take some time to build up to. It is so great for women, especially because, as I mentioned, the incidence of ACL injuries is higher in women than it is in men, so working on strengthening the legs with single-leg exercises will increase the strength and improve the tracking of the knee joint and decrease risk of injury. It's hard to feel sexy and fit when you're limping around with an injury. Let's avoid that at all costs and get your legs as strong as possible to be able to handle anything.

START: Stand on your right leg with a bench behind you. Extend your left leg forward so that the heel stays just off the floor at all times.

MOVEMENT: Bend your right leg and lower yourself to the bench. Do not sit down. Instead, skim the bench and then drive back up to the starting position. During the movement, be sure to keep your right knee tracking over your middle toe. Initially, your range will be limited, but as you get better at it over time, aim to increase your range of motion by removing the bench and using a squat rack or other stable object to hold onto for light support until you are able to perform a single leg squat with full range of motion. Use only your bodyweight to start.

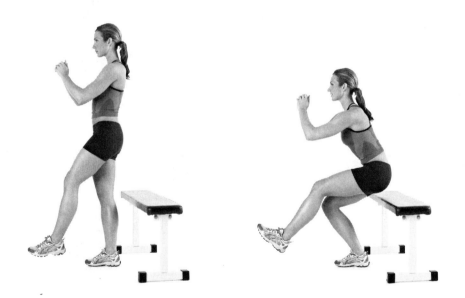

ALTERNATING LATERAL RAISE

Sculpt your shoulders while working your core—talk about bang for your buck!

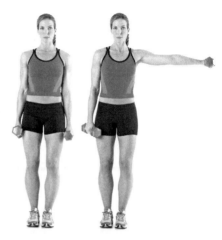

START: Stand with your feet shoulder-width apart and hold a dumbbell in each hand.

MOVEMENT: Brace your abs and lift one arm straight out to the side until it is straight out from the shoulder. Hold for a moment, then lower the arm under control. Alternate arms.

SUPINATED HIP EXTENSION WITH LEG CURL (SHELC)

There are only two exercises I know of that work both actions of the hamstrings, and this is one of them. Doing this exercise will really tone up the back of your legs and strengthen your "hammies."

START: Lie on the floor with your calves on a Swiss ball. Your arms should be out to your sides with your palms facing up.

MOVEMENT: Raise your hips until your body forms a straight line from your shoulders to your feet. From this position, keeping your hips in line with your shoulders and knees, bend your knees to curl the ball underneath you. Then straighten your legs again while still keeping your hips extended. Slowly lower your hips to the starting position.

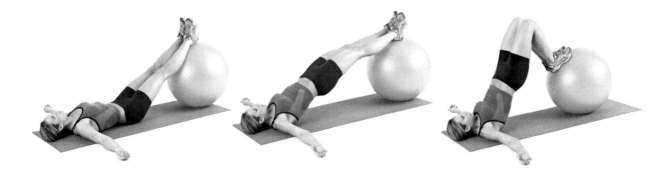

INVERTED ROW

This exercise, while focusing on working the muscles of the back in the rowing movement, is absolutely a total-body exercise. It's what I call a "bang for your buck" exercise. You'll feel your legs, your butt, your core, and your upper body working.

START: Lie on your back on the floor under an Olympic bar that is placed securely in a squat rack, at a height that's just slightly beyond arm's length. Your chest should be directly under the bar, and your legs should be straight. Grab the bar with an overhand grip and lift your hips, keeping your body in a straight line from head to ankles. The position looks like the starting position of an upside-down pushup. If this position is too difficult, bend your knees and put your feet flat on the floor to decrease the load by distributing more of your weight onto your legs.

MOVEMENT: Performing a rowing motion, pull your upper body up to the bar so that your chest touches the bar. Keep your body completely flat throughout the motion. Once the exercise becomes easy, you can increase the training effect by raising your feet onto a bench or, eventually, a Swiss ball.

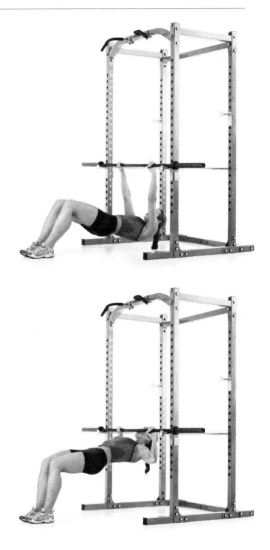

"Dial It In" Phase, Workout A

PLANK ON SWISS BALL

This is another example of taking an exercise through a progression. You did planks in a previous phase and strengthened your core while you learned to recruit the deep muscles of your transversus abdominis and pelvic floor. Now you'll take it up a notch by putting your elbows on a Swiss ball. As this gets easier, you can make it even more challenging by elevating your feet onto a step or bench.

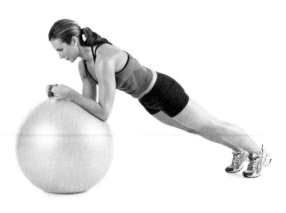

START: With your toes on the floor and your forearms on a Swiss ball, hold your body in a stable, straight line from shoulders to ankles. Keep your abs drawn in tight.

MOVEMENT: This is a static hold without any movement. Maintain your body in a straight line, keeping your core extremely tight.

UPPER-BODY CORE STABILITY RUSSIAN TWIST (See page 164)

DEADLIFT

There is nothing like deadlifts—just pure, raw lifting a weight off the floor. This exercise makes you feel like the empowered female that you are. You will work EVERYTHING. No joke, I can't think of what is not working, right down to your pinkie toes. This is one of the ultimate fit female exercises.

START: With a barbell on the floor (at a dead stop, hence the name), bend over, grasp the bar with an overhand grip, and place your shins against the bar, touching it. Bend your knees so that your thighs are slightly above parallel to the floor but keep your shoulders directly over your hands on the bar or, even better, slightly behind them. Keep your head in neutral alignment but look upward slightly.

MOVEMENT: Keeping an arch in your lower back (imperative, as rounding the lower back prevents these muscles from activating properly), pull the bar straight off the floor and bring your hips forward. The bar should never leave contact with your body. The uppermost position has you standing fully erect. Think about pushing the earth away from you, like a jumping action rather than a lifting action. Lower the bar under control to the floor (by flexing your hips and then your knees) to complete the repetition.

MILITARY PRESS

Build up your shoulders to make your hips appear smaller! Having toned, athletic shoulders changes your entire appearance. This move is an oldie but a goodie when it comes to strength training, and it still works. Because you're doing it standing, it becomes a core exercise, too. Any time you push a weight overhead, your core must switch on, so keep your abs tight.

START: Stand with a dumbbell in each hand at shoulder height, palms facing forward. Your knees should be slightly bent, not locked, and your abs should be engaged.

MOVEMENT: Extend your arms straight overhead and touch the dumbbells together at the top. Pause and lower the weights under control to the starting position.

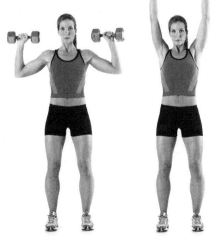

FORWARD AND BACK STEP-OVER

This exercise will make your leg burn, baby, burn, working your muscles not only as you lunge forward, but as you lunge backward as well. Again focus your vision on where you are going and how great you will look and feel to get you through the exercise without stopping.

START: Stand in a lunge position with your right foot on a step in front of you. Your body should be upright. You can start with body weight or holding light dumbbells.

MOVEMENT: Push off your left leg and step over the box to land in a lunge position with your left leg in front and your right foot still up on the step behind you. Push off your left foot again and return to the starting position. As you master this exercise, keep the leg on the step bent and under tension. The less your torso goes up and down, the harder and more effective the exercise will be. Perform eight repetitions going forward and back totaling 16 lunges on one leg. Then switch and repeat on the other leg.

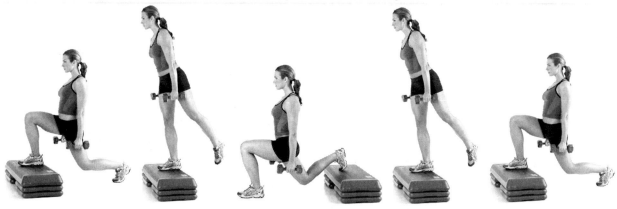

INCLINE DUMBBELL BENCH PRESS

Built-in Wonderbra! By strengthening the muscles under your breast tissue, you'll have a natural bra that will help keep things perky. This exercise will help tighten and tone the muscles that hold up your breasts. We must, we must, we must increase our bust. . . . Unfortunately, although this will help lift them, as you lose fat, your boobs will shrink. Sorry, ladies, I wish we could choose which part of your body will lose fat, but we can't.

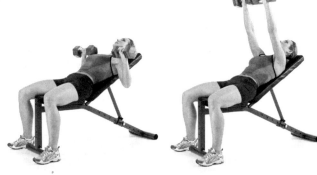

START: Lie on your back on a bench or a Swiss ball and hold a dumbbell in each hand near your shoulders, palms facing your feet.

MOVEMENT: Push the dumbbells straight up until your arms are fully extended, with the dumbbells nearly touching in this top position. Lower them to the starting position.

SINGLE-LEG SHELC

Doing this exercise with one leg will expose any imbalances between your two legs and help even them out. At the same time, increasing the instability of the basic exercise puts a greater demand on your core muscles.

START: Lie on your back with your left foot on a Swiss ball and your hands rotated out to the sides. Your right leg should be off the ball and in the air.

MOVEMENT: With only your left leg on the ball, raise your hips. From this position, keeping your hips extended, bend your left knee to curl the ball underneath you. Then straighten your left leg again while still keeping your hips extended. Slowly lower your hips to the starting position. Perform all of the reps on one leg and then switch legs and repeat.

ONE-POINT DUMBBELL ROW

In previous phases you did a three-point dumbbell row and a two-point dumbbell row, so in this phase we'll take it to the next progression, which is a one-point dumbbell row. Standing on one leg instead of two adds whole new challenges to this exercise, including balance, core recruitment, and all of your weight on one leg. As you are getting stronger, it's important to slowly increase the difficulty of your exercises to keep your body changing in response to new demands, and these three exercises are a perfect example of how to progress with each phase.

START: Stand on your right leg and bend over at the hip, holding one dumbbell straight down in your left hand. Your back should be flat with your spine in a straight line.

MOVEMENT: Squeeze your shoulder blades back and together to raise the dumbbell to your side in a rowing motion, then return the weight to the starting position. Maintain the position of your back throughout the movement, without coming up or rounding.

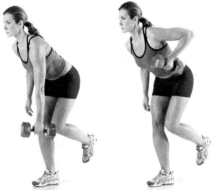

FINISHER: SQUAT THRUST AND TUCK JUMP OR BODY-WEIGHT SQUAT

Another finisher, to accomplish just that . . . finish you! Get ready!

This finisher involves squat thrusts in increments of three, done in supersets with tuck jumps or body-weight squats in single increments. Perform the following:

3 squat thrusts

1 tuck jump or body-weight squat

6 squat thrusts

2 tuck jumps or body-weight squats

9 squat thrusts

3 tuck jumps or body-weight squats

12 squat thrusts

4 tuck jumps or body-weight squats, etc.

FIT FEMALES USE RACKS

Part of becoming a fit female and getting comfortable in the gym is getting used to using a rack. There are a few exercises in the fit female program for which you'll need to use a rack. There are two reasons for this:

1. The amount of weight you can lift with your legs should be more than you could lift off the floor with your arms. If your biceps can lift it, it won't be enough to challenge your legs. As you are learning the technique of the squat and are increasing the weight you're using, you should place the bar in the rack at a height even with your shoulders. Load the bar with plates until the bar and plates together equal the amount you can lift. Walk up to the bar and, as we say in the gym, "address the bar." It might sound funny, but you do want to have respect for the weight you're about to lift and use proper form to lift the bar off the rack and place it on your body, to ensure that you don't injure yourself. I am a stickler about this in the gym, because being silly with a weight on your body is a great way to hurt yourself and end up injured and on the couch.

I don't want to scare you, because lifting weights is *extremely* safe as long as it's done properly. When you lift the weight off the rack, whether you're lifting it to do a front squat, a back squat, or a barbell lunge, you should place both feet under you, brace your core, and stand up straight with the weight.

Once the weight is on your body, DO NOT take a hand off to scratch something while balancing the bar on your back (I've seen people do this) and DO NOT twist around to take a look at who's watching you. Instead, keep your eyes straight ahead, stay focused on the exercise you're about to perform, and get it done. Complete the exercise, then walk straight back to set the weight down.

2. Using a rack, you can set yourself up with the safety bars so you can be confident that if you challenge yourself and get stuck, instead of losing your form and hurting yourself, you have the safety bars there to catch you. This way you can squat with confidence. The safety bars are the bars you see down lower in a rack. Adjust them to the appropriate height so that when you're at the bottom of your squat, the safety bars are just underneath the barbell, so you could easily set the bar on them and duck out from under it if for some reason you could not get yourself back up. For the most part, you should be increasing weights slowly enough so that you never get into this situation, but it is a good idea to use the safety bars in case you are having an off day. Plus, you'll definitely look like you know what you're doing in the gym when you start adjusting the bars in the rack.

Exercises with which to use a rack: Front squat, back squat, barbell split squat.

"Dial It In" Phase, Workout B

PRONE COBRA (See page 165)

FRONT SQUAT

Squats are one of the core fit female exercises, because they work pretty much everything, burn a ton of calories, and will challenge your body. Why a front squat and not a back squat? Front squats are an excellent exercise because you cannot cheat. With a back squat, most women have a tendency to round their backs and lose their form. During a front squat, you have to keep your posture upright or the bar will fall. If using a bar is uncomfortable, you can use a medicine ball or a kettlebell to get started. The type of load doesn't matter. The key is that it is loaded in front of you, so that your entire back has to work to keep your body upright. As you get the form right and increase your strength, you can conquer a back squat, too.

START: With your arms straight in front of you, walk up to the bar until the bar is touching your neck. Place the bar as high on your collarbone as comfortable. The bar will rest on your shoulders. Grip the bar with your hands as close to your shoulders as is comfortable and ensure that your elbows are pointing directly forward. The bar should be pressed against your throat. Stand with your feet shoulder-width apart and have your feet either straight or with the toes angled slightly outward. If you're uncomfortable using a bar, use a kettlebell instead.

MOVEMENT: Bend at the knees and hips to squat as deeply as you can, keeping your torso upright, then return to the starting position. The downward motion should exactly mirror the upward one. Keep your knees an equal distance apart throughout the movement, and keep your elbows up; don't let them sag. As you squat down, think about sending your elbows up to the ceiling to keep a good position.

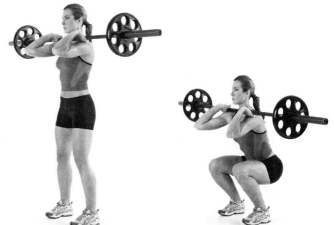

CHINUP (See page 175)

ROMANIAN DEADLIFT

Having a nicely shaped butt is part of what defines a fit female in my mind. Only athletes and women who work out have butts that are made up of muscle, look good in jeans, and are not flat, saggy, or jiggly. It takes hard work to build a nice-looking butt. There are many exercises in this routine that target your butt for this reason—to give you a fit female derriere! If you don't want a butt, this program is not for you. The Romanian deadlift is another great move for your entire derriere, including your hamstrings, glutes, and lower back.

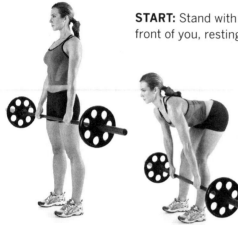

START: Stand with your feet shoulder-width apart and hold a barbell in front of you, resting on your thighs.

MOVEMENT: Kicking your hips back and keeping the bar right along your legs, lower the bar until you feel a stretch in your hamstrings, but be sure to maintain a neutral spine. Do not round your back. Keep your knees slightly bent, not locked. Return to the starting position.

DUMBBELL PUSH PRESS

More bang for your buck! This exercise looks like an upper-body exercise, but you are actually lifting a weight that you need to use your lower body to explode up and lift. And as the weight lands overhead, your core must switch on to support it. So your upper body, lower body, and core will all benefit. And you'll feel your heart pumping from the explosive movement. This is great for getting your metabolism revving.

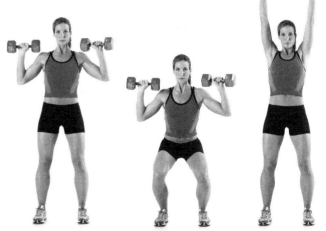

START: Stand holding two dumbbells at your shoulders.

MOVEMENT: Using the momentum from your legs, start with a small bend of your knees and then explode upward as you push the dumbbells overhead. This is an explosive movement and should be done with a weight that you could not simply press up with your arms alone. Pause with the weights overhead, then return them to the starting position.

BARBELL SPLIT SQUAT

Show off those legs! Picture yourself wearing a miniskirt or short shorts that reveal your lean, defined legs, and not having to worry about cellulite or anything jiggling. This exercise in particular hits your legs a little differently than a lunge, even though it looks very similar to a lunge. The split squat action is actually more a movement of the front leg, letting your knee move forward, tracking directly over your toe, and then driving back through the glute, making the motion more hip dominant. A lunge is more of an up-and-down motion that uses more quad strength. These are both great exercises, and both are used throughout this program to give you legs you can feel confident showing off!

START: Standing with a barbell on your back, your chest up tall, your stomach tight, and your feet shoulder-width apart, step forward about three feet with your right leg.

MOVEMENT: Bend your right knee and lower yourself into a lunge position, keeping your right heel down the entire time. Your left knee will bend, too, as you lower yourself, but most of the movement is in the front leg. Your right thigh should be in contact with your right calf at the bottom of the movement. Think about having a walnut between your thigh and calf, and you need to crack the nut. Once in the bottom position, concentrate on recruiting your right glute and leg to drive through your right leg and return to the starting position.

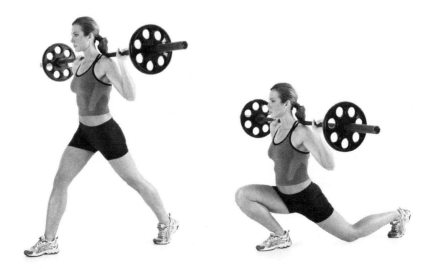

SPLIT-STANCE SINGLE-ARM CABLE ROW

In the base phase, you performed this exercise using two arms at once. By now, your back should be getting strong, and you should have better posture than when you started. Using one arm instead of two creates more of a transverse motion, allowing you to recruit more of your core muscles.

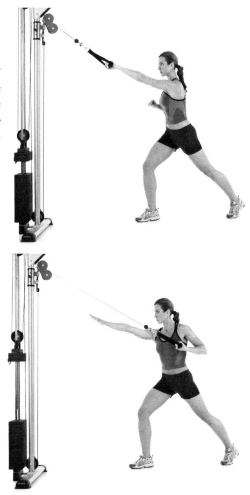

START: Stand facing a high cable pulley with one handle attached and position your legs in a split stance, with your left foot in front of your right. Grasp the handle with your right hand and position your body so your right arm is extended and the weight is lifted just off the stack to start.

MOVEMENT: Using your back muscles, pull your right shoulder blade in toward your spine, letting your elbow bend as you row the cable toward your body. Keep your elbow in close to you and your shoulder down. Pull the handle in as far as you can while still maintaining your form. Pause, then resist the load as you slowly extend your arm to return the handle to the starting position.

FINISHER: LEG MATRIX

At our gym, this is known as torture, screamers, and "that insane leg thing," among other names. It is challenging, but it will accomplish the goal of finishing you off.

All in a row, without stopping, perform the following:

20 body-weight squats

20 body-weight dynamic lunges on alternating legs

20 lunge jumps

20 jump squats

Time yourself and try to beat your time each week.

Fine-tune Phase, Workout A

PLANK WITH ALTERNATE ARM REACH

This is another progression from a previous exercise. You've done planks on the floor and planks on a Swiss ball, and now we'll go back to the floor and progress by adding a reach. There are so many different ways to perform this exercise. This will take your core training to the next level.

START: Once on the floor, support your full weight on your forearms and toes.

MOVEMENT: Just like you did with the Bird Dog in the Base Phase, lift your right arm and left leg straight out, extending your arm and lifting it so it's in line with your ear. Keep your core as still and stable as possible. Return to the starting position and repeat on the opposite side.

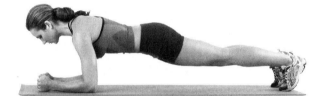

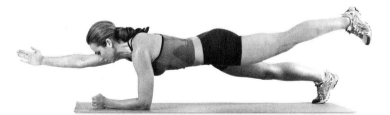

COMPLEX

A barbell complex can be defined as two or more movements performed in a sequence without rest, using the same load. Each movement is performed for a given number of repetitions before going on to the next movement. The complex is completed when all the prescribed repetitions of each movement are finished. The advantage of this type of training is obvious—in a short period of time, in a limited space, with limited equipment, you can get a lot accomplished. The metabolic effect of this type of work is unparalleled—you get increased work demand, use more muscle groups, increase work capacity, and massively boost caloric expenditure.

START: Holding dumbbells, a standard bar, or a lighter bar, stand with your feet shoulder-width apart. Use a lighter weight for these complexes than you would for the individual exercises in the complex. You'll hold the weight throughout the complex without setting it down.

MOVEMENT: Perform the following exercises in sequence without stopping.

DEADLIFT: Bend your knees and touch the bar to the floor, then stand back up. Do 8 repetitions.

HIGH PULL: Without letting go of the bar, stand upright with a slight bend at your waist and bend your knees. Then explode upward as if you were going to jump, and create enough momentum so that the bar comes up to chest height, with your elbows bending out.

PUSH PRESS: Bend your legs slightly, then use them to help you explode the bar up overhead. Return it to the front of your body, then lift it overhead again for 8 repetitions. You're finished!

REVERSE LUNGE: Standing upright, with the bar still on your shoulders, step backward with your right leg into a reverse lunge. Alternate legs until you've completed 8 repetitions with each leg.

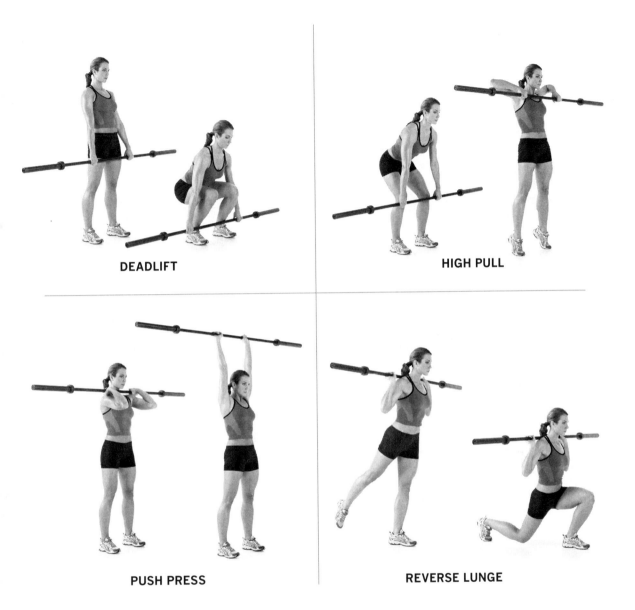

DEADLIFT

HIGH PULL

PUSH PRESS

REVERSE LUNGE

BULGARIAN SPLIT DEADLIFT

There's nothing like taking a really challenging, supereffective exercise up another notch, which is exactly what we're doing here. This exercise turns the Bulgarian split squat into a more hip-dominant exercise. Again, ladies, you are building a fit, powerful, sexy butt! Any time you put the weight in front of you, you have to recruit more of your glutes and hamstrings.

START: Stand with a bench behind you and hold dumbbells in your hands. Facing away from the bench, place your left foot on the bench and your right foot two to three feet in front of the bench. You'll be in a modified lunge position except different from the last time you did Bulgarian split squats. Your torso will be bending forward to lift and lower the weights using more hips.

MOVEMENT: With the bulk of your body weight on your right leg, bend your right knee until your right thigh is below parallel to the floor and the knee of your left leg is grazing the floor. At the same time, bend forward at the waist to touch the dumbbells to the floor, keeping your weight on your right leg. (Do not sit back and put weight on your left leg. That is cheating!) Pause in this position, then return to a fully upright stance. Repeat for the desired number of reps, then switch sides. Do not just bend over at the hips and touch the weights to the floor. You must bend your knees and only bend at the hips as much as you need to. Your back should not round but should stay neutral so you're using your legs and hips, not your back, to move the weights.

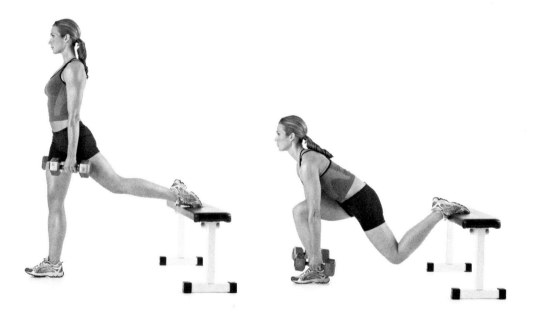

SINGLE-ARM DUMBBELL CHEST PRESS ON SWISS BALL

This is another progression from a previous exercise. Any time you add an unstable object to the mix, you're challenging your body in a different way. You can change it up even more by alternating your arms. Performing a dumbbell chest press on a Swiss ball invites a whole new set of muscles to the party. On the ball, you'll feel your abs and your legs working, along with your shoulders, triceps, and chest. Be sure you have a strong Swiss ball that can handle your body weight along with that of some dumbbells. Be careful, because some gyms buy cheap Swiss balls that are meant for kids to play with in the backyard, not for you to lie on while balancing heavy weights. Search the surface of the ball for a weight-limit notation stating how much it can handle. You shouldn't decrease the amount of weight you use just because you're on a ball. You've gained a lot of strength, so be sure to push yourself and lift enough weight to challenge yourself. Being on a ball doesn't make it a foofy, girly exercise.

START: Lie on a Swiss ball (you can also use a BOSU balance trainer, which is like half of a Swiss ball) with your hips level with your shoulders so that you're on an incline. Hold one dumbbell and push it straight up so your arms are extended.

MOVEMENT: Lower the dumbbell, then press it back up. The entire time you'll have to keep your abs tight, your butt engaged, and your legs working to keep you balanced on the ball.

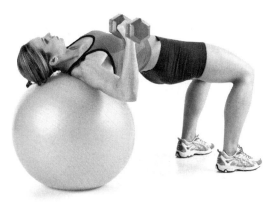

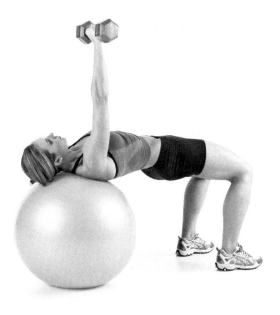

BACK SQUAT

You conquered the front squat in an earlier phase. Now it's time to master the back squat. Squats are a huge part of a fit female's program because they work all the muscles of your legs along with your abs, and they burn a ton of calories. We use several variations of squats throughout this program, including the back squat. This is just one variation of an extremely effective exercise for building the fit, sexy body you want.

START: With a barbell as high on your neck as is comfortable, grip the bar with your hands as close to your shoulders as you can. Be sure that your elbows are pointing directly down toward the floor. Your feet should be shoulder-width apart and either oriented straight ahead or rotated outward slightly.

MOVEMENT: Bending at the knees and hips, squat as deeply as you can, keeping your torso upright. (Think about keeping your chest up as if you have a string pulling up your chest.) Then return to the starting position. The upward movement should exactly mirror the downward movement. Your knees should stay the same distance apart throughout the move. If they collapse inward, decrease the weight you're using and think about squeezing your butt muscles as you do the exercise.

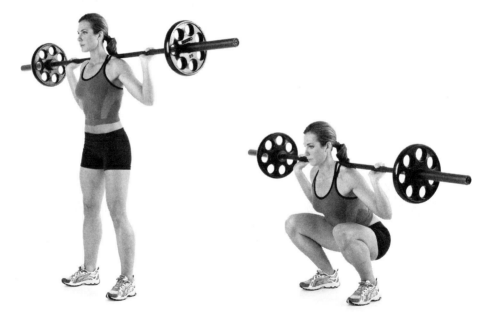

CHINUP (See page 181)

Fine-tune Phase, Workout B

SWISS BALL CRUNCH

If you're going to do crunches, do not do them for 500 reps on the floor! Abdominal muscles are like any other muscle. They need to be loaded to be built up enough to see them, and they need to be worked in their full range of motion. By doing them on a Swiss ball, you can extend your torso all the way to get the full range of motion before performing the crunching movement. This is the only crunch I have in this entire book. Every other core exercise is about stability, and, really, so is this one.

START: Lie face up on a Swiss ball, with your navel at the apex of the ball. Place your hands behind your head and your tongue against the roof of your mouth. (This is the anatomical rest position for the tongue. Believe it or not, doing this will eliminate the neck strain most people feel, while also making you stronger.)

MOVEMENT: From this position, curl your torso up, one vertebra at a time, until you're fully contracted. Focus on bringing your rib cage and hips closer together. In this contracted position, pause, then reverse the motion. Concentrate on moving one vertebra at a time until you're in the fully stretched position. Once you're strong enough, you can add weight in the form of a dumbbell on your chest, to really create those abs of steel.

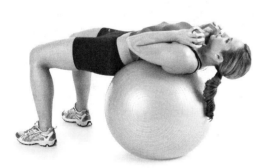
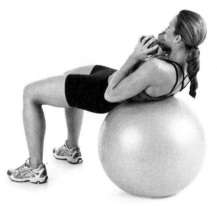

COMPLEX

On day two, you'll do exactly as you did on day one, but with different exercises.

START: Holding dumbbells, a standard bar, or a lighter bar, stand with your feet shoulder-width apart. Use a lighter weight for this complex than you would for the individual exercises in it. You'll hold the weight throughout the complex without setting it down.

MOVEMENT: Perform the following exercises in sequence without stopping.

HIGH PULL: Stand upright with a slight bend at your waist and bend in your knees. Then explode upward as if you were going to jump, and create enough momentum so that the bar comes up to chest height, with your elbows bending out. Do not lift the bar with your arms. It should come up as a result of the force you create.

FRONT SQUAT WITH PUSH PRESS: Holding the weight on the front of your shoulders with your elbows up and your torso extended, lower yourself into a squat. Then, as you're coming up from the bottom position, drive the bar up overhead into a push press. Carefully lower the bar to your shoulders and repeat. On the 8th rep, bring the bar behind your neck instead, in position for a back squat.

BACK SQUAT: With the bar on your back, chest up tall, and feet shoulder-width apart, lower yourself into a squat, then return to standing. Do 8 reps.

GOOD MORNING: Finish this complex with a good morning. Bend at the hips, stick your hips back, and stretch your hamstrings while the bar is on your back. This is very similar to a Romanian deadlift except that the bar is on your back instead of in front of you. Your weight should be on your heels, and your knees should not be locked. Go only as low as you can while maintaining a neutral spine. If your back starts to round, you've gone too far; stop and reverse the movement. Do 8 reps.

DEADLIFT (See page 183)

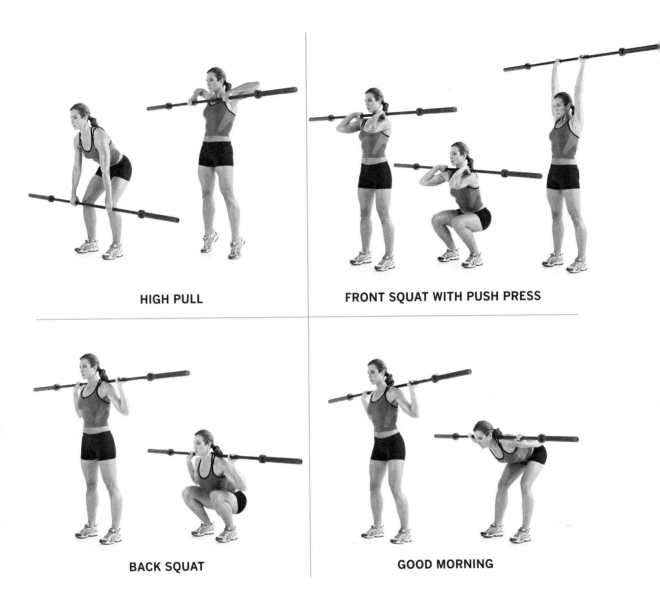

HIGH PULL

FRONT SQUAT WITH PUSH PRESS

BACK SQUAT

GOOD MORNING

DUMBBELL ROTATIONAL OVERHEAD PRESS

Take a traditional exercise like the military press and add a twist into the mix, and what do you have? A great exercise for toning the upper body, core, and legs. Your shoulders are working to press the weight overhead one at a time. Your core is on maximal recruitment, thanks to the twisting action and the weight overhead. Remember, anytime a weight goes overhead, your core has to work. Your legs are also getting in on the action because of the twisting motion to each side.

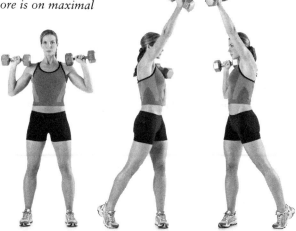

START: Stand with your feet shoulder-width apart and hold two dumbbells at your shoulders.

MOVEMENT: Press one dumbbell up overhead as you rotate your body. Return to the starting position and repeat on the opposite side. Rotate back and forth, pressing one arm, then the other, overhead.

SINGLE-LEG SQUAT (See page 179)

BENT-OVER ROW

This exercise allows you to take some of the strength you've built and use both arms, along with your back, glutes, and legs, to hold a load that will challenge you. As you are performing the bent-over row, your glutes and hamstrings will be contracting to keep you in position. Why so much rowing, you ask? Of course, to improve your posture, but also, all these rowing exercises will eliminate ever worrying about putting on a bra and having bra overhang. No more ugly bra fat! From now on, you will feel sexy in a bra and will look forward to both bra and bathing suit shopping, because you'll feel toned and confident in both. Start rowing!

START: Grab a bar with an underhand grip just outside shoulder width. Bend forward until your torso is parallel to the floor, so gravity will be working against you.

MOVEMENT: Using your back, pull your shoulder blades back and toward each other and bend your arms to bring the bar to your abdominals and your elbows to your sides. Pause, then return to the starting position. Be careful not to let your shoulders become tense. Also, as you get tired, you'll find your torso sneaking up; to keep an eye on this, stand with a mirror at your side.

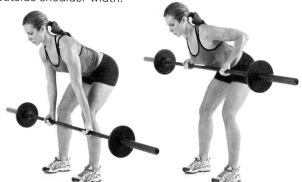

METABOLIC CIRCUITS

The following circuits are your cardio workouts. *Cardio* (short for *cardiovascular*) refers to any exercise in which your heart and lungs are involved. The word *aerobic,* on the other hand, denotes a state or intensity at which you do your cardio. All aerobic exercise is cardio, but not all cardio is aerobic. This program will use only nonaerobic, high-intensity cardio. You can achieve this on a treadmill or bike, increasing your heart rate for a one- to two-minute period and then recovering. However, in this program we're taking it one step further and challenging not only your heart and lungs but also the rest of your body with new movements, different planes of motion, and athletic exercises. These cardio workouts are the most effective for increasing your metabolism, creating an afterburn effect to burn more calories for the next 24 to 48 hours, and keeping your body changing to become a fit female.

These workouts are done interval-style. Your heart rate will increase, and then you'll recover and repeat. In each circuit, you should push yourself to the point where you cannot carry on a conversation. Set yourself up in front of a clock or with a stopwatch and go as hard as you can for the prescribed period of time. The beauty of this is that as you improve, the work intervals can get harder and harder, and the recovery intervals can be shortened, or performed at a higher speed. In fact, there is no limit and no downside to interval training. Push yourself to do more reps in the same amount of time each workout. Each phase, you'll either increase the frequency with which you do these workouts or increase the volume within each workout. It's all planned out for you.

I know what you're thinking . . . you don't want to look silly doing these. You'd rather stick to the treadmill, looking cool, strutting your stuff. Well, take a look at the treadmills at your gym and tell me if *anyone* walking on those treadmills has the body you want. I can bet that most of them have not changed their bodies in the three years they've been trudging on those treadmills every single morning, walking to nowhere. Most of them probably look flabby, have no definition, and have not changed their bodies one bit. And they probably don't look so cool and aren't necessarily strutting, but are doing the treadmill shuffle and looking miserable. To make a change, you have to do something different. I bet none of them look like the fit female you are becoming.

So get over worrying about what other people think of your workouts. Instead, stay focused on how hot you'll look and how good you'll feel at the end of the 16 weeks. You are a fit female, and fit females don't walk on treadmills. Besides, I bet as your body is changing and everyone at your gym sees you doing these workouts, you'll be bombarded with questions on what you're doing. You will become the expert, because you are a fit female inspiring others! Pretty soon the treadmills will be empty, because everyone will be following your lead.

You could also do these workouts at home, since no equipment is needed, and save the gym for your strength-training workouts.

Choose one exercise from each of the Metabolic Exercise Groups for each of the two circuits. Whichever eight exercises you choose for the first phase, stick with them for 4 weeks and then switch to a different set of eight. Each time you do the workout, try to do more repetitions of each exercise in the same length of time.

THE METABOLIC MENU

Metabolic Exercise Group 1: Locomotion

Hop Scotch

Lateral Ski Jump

Lateral Step-Out Squat Moving

Rope Jumping

Sprint Run

Walking Lunges

Over/Under

Metabolic Exercise Group 2: Change of Levels—Unilateral

Single Leg Squat Thrusts

Cross Behind Step Up and Over

Explosive Step Up

Alternating Step Up

Lunge with Overhead Reach

Lunge Jumps

Metabolic Exercise Group 3: Core

Mountain Climber

Prone Cross Toe Touch

Prone Step Off on Swiss Ball

Medicine Ball Toss

Pushups

Spider Man

Metabolic Exercise Group 4: Change of Levels—Bilateral

Body-weight Squat

Body-weight Jump Squat

Squat Thrusts

Static Squat In-and-Out Jump

Kettlebell or Dumbbell Single-Arm Clean

Kettlebell or Dumbbell Swing

Box Jump

Metabolic Circuit

You won't do these circuits in weeks one and two; instead, you'll focus on your strength workouts. Then begin incorporating the metabolic circuits in week three, as shown here.

EXERCISE	WEEK	ROUNDS	TIME	REST
Metabolic 1A Exercise Group 1	3–4	1–2	30 seconds	30 seconds
	5–8	2–3	30 seconds	15 seconds
	9–12	2–3	45 seconds	10 seconds
	13–16	3–4	60 seconds	0 seconds
Metabolic 1B Exercise Group 2	3–4	1–2	30 seconds	90 seconds
	5–8	2–3	30 seconds	60 seconds
	9–12	2–3	45 seconds	60 seconds
	13–16	3–4	60 seconds	30 seconds
Metabolic 1C Exercise Group 3	3–4	1–2	30 seconds	30 seconds
	5–8	2–3	30 seconds	15 seconds
	9–12	2–3	45 seconds	10 seconds
	13–16	3–4	60 seconds	0 seconds
Metabolic 1D Exercise Group 4	3–4	1–2	30 seconds	90 seconds
	5–8	2–3	30 seconds	60 seconds
	9–12	2–3	45 seconds	60 seconds
	13–16	3–4	60 seconds	30 seconds
Metabolic 2A Exercise Group 1	3–4	1–2	30 seconds	30 seconds
	5–8	2–3	30 seconds	15 seconds
	9–12	2–3	45 seconds	10 seconds
	13–16	3–4	60 seconds	0 seconds
Metabolic 2B Exercise Group 2	3–4	1–2	30 seconds	2 minutes
	5–8	2–3	30 seconds	90 seconds
	9–12	2–3	45 seconds	90 seconds
	13–16	3–4	60 seconds	1 minute
Metabolic 2C Exercise Group 3	3–4	1–2	30 seconds	30 seconds
	5–8	2–3	30 seconds	15 seconds
	9–12	2–3	45 seconds	10 seconds
	13–16	3–4	60 seconds	0 seconds
Metabolic 2D Exercise Group 4	3–4	1–2	30 seconds	2 minutes
	5–8	2–3	30 seconds	90 seconds
	9–12	2–3	45 seconds	90 seconds
	13–16	3–4	60 seconds	1 minute

EXERCISE DESCRIPTIONS
FOR METABOLIC CIRCUITS
Metabolic Exercise Group 1—Locomotion

HOPSCOTCH

START: Stand with your feet wider than shoulder-width apart.

MOVEMENT: Think back to hopscotch days. Jump forward and bring your feet together, then jump forward again and land with your feet apart. From there, jump backward, bringing your feet together again, and then back to the starting position.

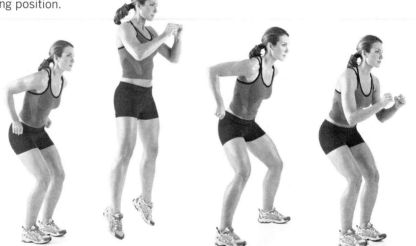

LATERAL SKI JUMP

START: Stand on your right leg.

MOVEMENT: Push off your right leg to jump to the left and land on your left leg. Then jump to the right, landing on your right leg. Keep your knees bent and jump as far as you can back and forth. You should feel like an inline skater.

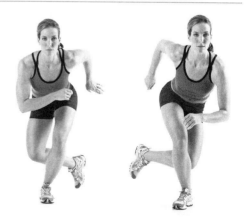

LATERAL STEP-OUT SQUAT

START: Stand with your feet together and your knees bent at least 90 degrees.

MOVEMENT: Step out to one side into a squat, maintaining the same knee bend or deeper. Return to the starting position, then step out to the other side. Repeat back and forth for the prescribed time period.

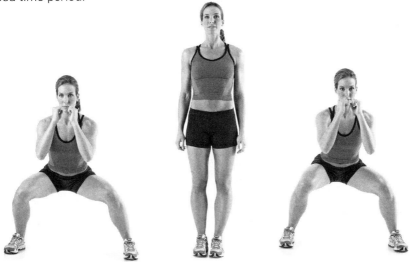

ROPE JUMPING

START: If you have a jump rope, use it. If not, pretend. Stand with the rope's ends in your hands.

MOVEMENT: Jump rope! Vary your jumps: two feet, one foot at a time, high knees. Stay on your toes, with your knees bent.

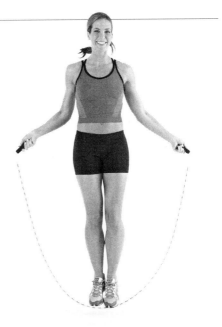

SPRINT RUN

START: Stand in a room large enough to run back and forth in, or with an object you can run around in a circle, such as a barbell.

MOVEMENT: Run back and forth or around the object for the allotted time. Sprint and change directions as fast as you can to get your heart rate pumping.

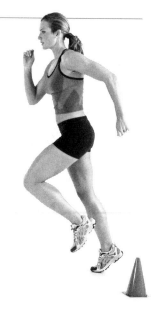

WALKING LUNGES

START: Stand with your feet together.

MOVEMENT: Step out into a lunge with your left leg keeping your posture upright. As you come up from the lunge position putting your weight on the left leg bring your right leg up and through to the front stepping in to a lunge with your right foot. Continued alternating legs as you are lunge walking forward.

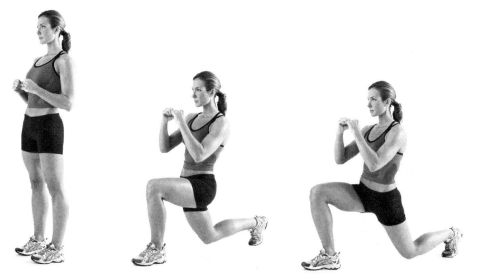

OVER/UNDER

START: Stand with your feet shoulder-width apart and imagine there's a stick placed horizontally in front of you at waist height.

MOVEMENT: Lift your right leg over the imaginary stick from left to right, then duck under, coming back the other direction, from right to left.

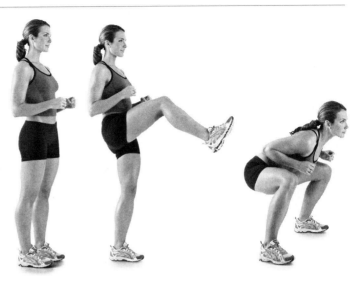

SPLIT JACK

START: Stand with your arms at your sides.

MOVEMENT: Jump and land with your left foot in front of you and your right foot behind. At the same time, with straight arms, swing your left arm forward toward your right leg. Then jump again, switching arms and legs. This is very similar to a jumping jack, except the motion is front to back instead of out to the sides.

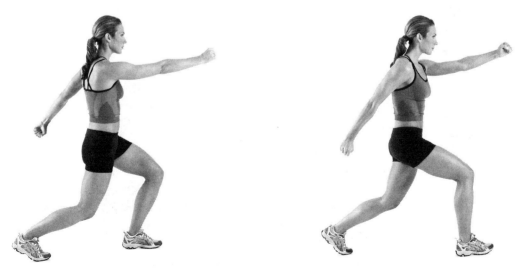

Metabolic Exercise Group 2—Change of Levels Unilateral

SINGLE-LEG ALTERNATING SQUAT THRUST

START: Stand on your right leg with your arms at your sides.

MOVEMENT: Bend down and touch the floor with both hands, keeping all your weight on your right leg. Then jump out into a one-legged pushup position on your right foot, jump back in, and stand up. Alternate legs.

CROSS-BEHIND STEPUP AND OVER

START: Stand with a bench or step at your right side and place your right foot on the bench.

MOVEMENT: Drive through your right leg and stand up on the bench. Cross your left leg behind you and land on the opposite side of the step, keeping your right leg on the bench the entire time. From there, drive through your right leg again to stand back up on the bench and bring your left leg back through to end in the starting position. Go back and forth for half the allotted time, then switch sides and repeat.

EXPLOSIVE STEPUP

START: Stand with a low step in front of you and your right foot on the step.

MOVEMENT: Put your weight on your right foot on the step. Explode off as you switch legs.

BODY-WEIGHT ALTERNATING STEPUP

START: Stand with a step in front of you.

MOVEMENT: This will take you back to step class, except the difference is that you won't be doing it for an hour. Instead, the goal is to get your heart rate up for 30 seconds to two minutes and push the intensity. Step up on the step with one foot, then the other, and then back down. Alternate which foot you step up with first on each repetition.

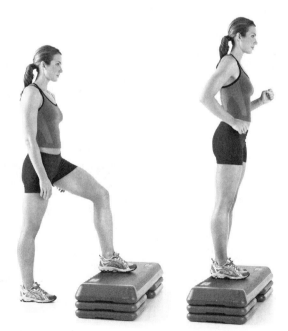

DYNAMIC LUNGE WITH OVERHEAD REACH

START: Stand with your feet shoulder-width apart and hold either a medicine ball or simply use arms to reach up wihout holding anything.

MOVEMENT: Step forward into a lunge with your left leg while you life the ball overhead with straight arms until your arms are in line with your ears. You'll finish in a full lunge position with your arms extended overhead. From this position, think about driving through the heel of your left leg and using your leg and glutes to push off and back to the starting position. Alternate legs.

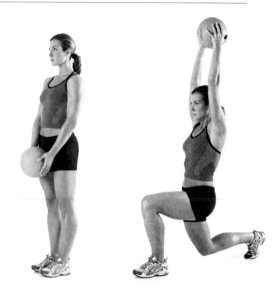

LUNGE JUMPS

START: In a lunge position with your left leg in front.

MOVEMENT: Drive off both legs exploding into the air and mid air switch legs and land in a lunge with your right foot in front. Repeat alternating back and forth for the time period.

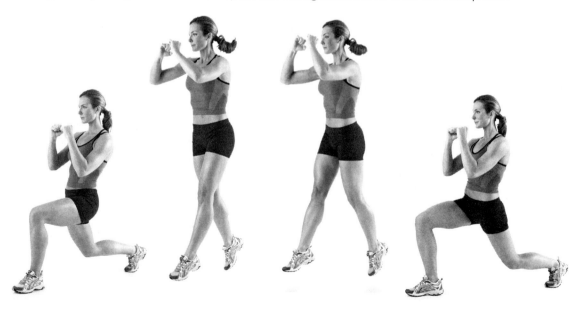

Metabolic Exercise Group 3—Core

MOUNTAIN CLIMBER

START: Assume a standard pushup position.

MOVEMENT: Drive one knee up toward your chest, then return the leg to the starting position as you bring the other knee toward your chest. Alternate legs as fast as possible.

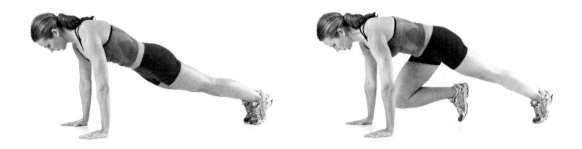

PRONE CROSS-TOE TOUCH

START: Assume a standard pushup position.

MOVEMENT: Cross your right leg under your body and touch your foot to your left hand, then return the foot to the starting position. Now cross your left foot under your body to touch your right hand, then return. Continue to alternate legs.

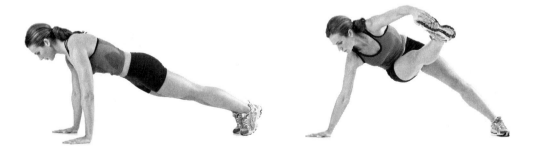

PRONE STEP-OFF ON SWISS BALL

START: Assume a pushup position with your feet on a Swiss ball.

MOVEMENT: Maintain your body position and keep your legs straight as you lift your right foot off the ball and touch it to the floor beside the ball. Bring your right foot back onto the ball and repeat with your left leg. Continue to alternate legs.

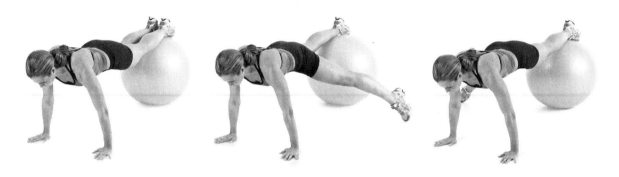

MEDICINE BALL TOSS

START: Stand holding a medicine ball in both hands.

MOVEMENT: Lift the medicine ball overhead and then, as hard as you can, using your whole body (legs, abs, everything), slam the ball against the floor. Be careful it doesn't bounce up and hit you in the face. Catch the ball and repeat.

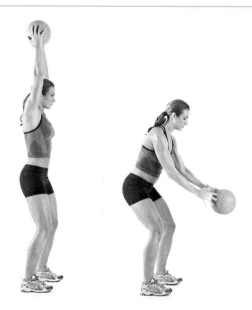

PUSHUPS

START: In a pushup position.

MOVEMENT: Perform a pushup by bending your elbows until they are in line with your shoulders. Keep your stomach tight. Push the ground away from you to return to the start position. Perform as many reps as you can get in the time period. Do not use pushups in your metabolic workout until you are strong enough to do them with your body weight for 10-15 repetitions without getting sore. You will get to the point where pushups can be part of your metabolic cardio workout.

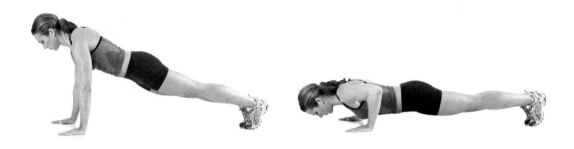

SPIDER MAN

START: Assume a standard pushup position.

MOVEMENT: Explode off the floor and land with your right hand reaching out beyond your head, your right leg straight back, and your left hand and foot next to each other, as if you were Spider Man climbing a wall. Explode and switch to the exact opposite position. Continue to alternate.

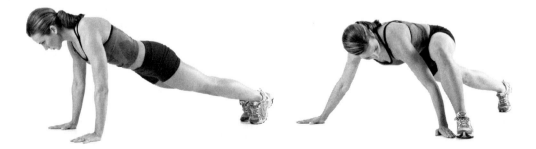

Metabolic Exercise Group 4—Change of Levels, Bilateral

BODY-WEIGHT SQUAT

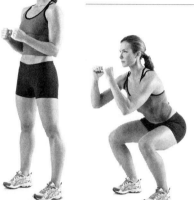

START: Stand with your feet shoulder-width apart and your arms at your sides.

MOVEMENT: Squat until your thighs are at or below parallel to the floor, return to the starting position, and repeat. Keep your knees tracking over your toes and keep your heels down the entire time.

BODY-WEIGHT JUMP SQUAT

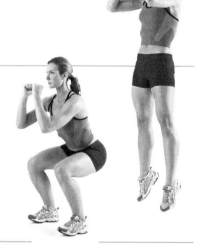

START: In a squat position.

MOVEMENT: Push the ground away from you and jump as high as you can off the floor. Land back in a squat position and repeat.

SQUAT THRUST

START: Stand with your feet together and your arms   at your sides.

MOVEMENT: Bend down and touch the floor with your hands. Put weight on your hands and jump out so your legs are extended into a pushup position, then jump back in so your feet are at your hands again and stand up.

To make it more advanced, add a vertical jump at the end.

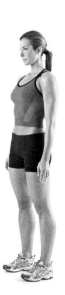

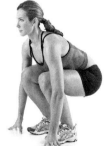

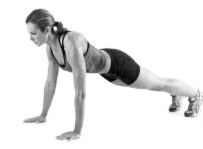

STATIC SQUAT IN-AND-OUT JUMP

START: Stand with your legs together and knees bent.

MOVEMENT: Keeping your knees bent and staying low, jump out into a wide squat and back in.

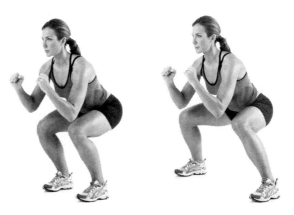

KETTLEBELL OR DUMBBELL SINGLE-ARM CLEAN

START: Stand with the weight on the floor between your legs.

MOVEMENT: Bend down to pick up the weight with one hand and, using your hips and legs, lift the weight up to the front squat position, with your arm and wrist locked straight. Bend your knees and lower the weight back to the floor. For the next rep, lift the weight with your other hand, and continue to alternate sides.

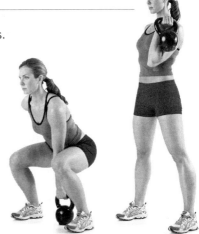

KETTLEBELL OR DUMBBELL SWING

I love using kettlebells for an excellent metabolic workout, but learning all the fundamentals of training with kettlebells is a book in itself. For the purposes of this book, I want to introduce you to two exercises that you can add to your workouts to really challenge yourself. This can be done with a dumbbell just as effectively.

START: Stand with a kettlebell or dumbbell in both hands, with your feet in a wide-stance squat and the weight hanging between your legs.

MOVEMENT: The key with this exercise is to use your hips and legs, not your back or arms, to get the momentum going to swing the weight. Your body weight should be back on your heels, and as you bend your legs, sit back to switch on your glutes. Then, as you come up, think about thrusting your hips forward to swing the weight up. The weight should swing only to chest height. If it's going higher than chest height, grab a heavier weight.

BOX JUMP

START: Stand with a bench in front of you.

MOVEMENT: Jump with both feet onto the bench, then step back down. Repeat.

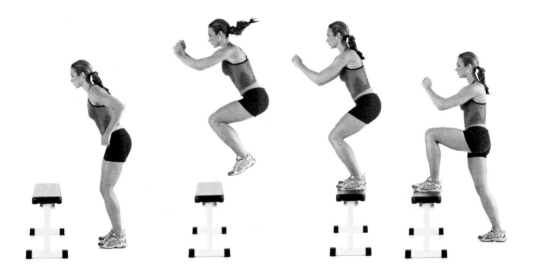

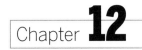
Fit Female Recovery and Regeneration Rituals

As you increase your exercise volume and work out more, you also need to give back to your body by making certain recovery and regeneration rituals a part of your repertoire. Remember Fit Female Credo Secret #7: Make R, R, & R a priority. You do not get the results from the workout itself; you get results from recovering from the workout. You're working out like an athlete, so you need to employ recovery techniques like an athlete. Most of us get an occasional massage for a special occasion, but it might be once a year at most. This is not enough when you're challenging your body on a weekly basis. Most professional athletes have a masseuse on hand as well as a nutritionist, and some even have professional stretchers. Well, of course I realize we can't all hire our own masseuse, nutritionist, and stretcher (wouldn't it be nice!), so we have to do the next best thing, which is just as effective, even if it's not as luxurious.

FIT FEMALE RITUALS

1. Shut-eye. Make sure you get seven to eight hours of sleep a night. Sleep is when your body repairs itself, and lack of sleep can wreak havoc on your body fat and your hormones. Establish a nightly ritual of doing something relaxing, such as taking a hot bath and doing your foam rolling and stretching, and then hit the sack at the same time every night and sleep for seven to eight hours a night consistently. People who sleep more weigh less. A study was done recently at Stanford University in which 1,000 volunteers reported the number of hours they slept each night. The people who got less than eight hours of sleep a night had higher body fat levels. Hit the sack for seven to eight hours a night to be a fit female!

"With the new day comes new strength and new thoughts."

—ELEANOR ROOSEVELT

2. Postworkout recovery shakes. Another ritual to add to your repertoire is to immediately drink a shake when you finish each workout. You must replace what you've depleted. Do not dillydally; instead, have your shake ready to go for immediate replenishment. You won't get everything out of your workout if you skip this step. You have to replenish your body immediately after your workout with quick-releasing carbohydrates and protein (a shake is best when it contains 60 to 80 grams of carbs and 15 to 20 grams of whey protein) to ensure optimal recovery. Don't be afraid of carbohydrates, especially when it comes to postworkout refueling. It's been shown in recent research studies that consuming a shake made up of a four-to-one ratio of carbohydrates to protein within 30 minutes of a workout will offset muscle damage and facilitate greater training adaptations. Make this a postworkout ritual.

3. Foam rolling. Throughout this program I want you to use something called a foam roller—a round cylinder of foam that you use to massage your muscles. This will loosen up anything that is becoming tight from your workouts (or from life) and get rid of any knots or adhesions. Adhesions are scar tissues in your muscles that keep them from performing optimally and could lead to injuries. When you first use a foam roller, you might not like it, because your muscles will probably feel very sore and the process might actually be a little tough to take the first few times around, because of knots in your muscles. Keep in mind that if you do have sore spots, this foam roller will really help: Healthy tissue shouldn't be painful, so if you have sore spots, it means there are adhesions or tightness that you need to get rid of. We want your muscle tissue to be as healthy as possible so that you can get the most out of your workouts. By rolling out these sore spots, you'll decrease the tension and eliminate the sore spots. Eventually, you won't be able to live without your foam roller, because your body will feel so much better when you're using it consistently.

4. Stretching. I know. "Stretching. *Boring!* Stretching doesn't get me lean and fit. Sweating and working hard does, not stretching. What a waste of time!" Well, hold on. The techniques in this chapter are not optional; they are part of the program. Make them part of your daily ritual.

I have news for you: If you don't stretch and foam roll, your muscles will not be able to work as hard as they might if you did, and you will not get the most out of your workouts. Can you imagine if spending an extra 10 minutes a day stretching and foam rolling improved the effectiveness of your workouts by, let's say, just 1 percent? When you're doing three workouts a week, every week, that is 12 percent a month in increased benefit from your workouts. Do you think that will have an effect on your results? Uhhh, yeah!

Plus, foam rolling and stretching is an easy way to perk up your posture and make yourself look as if you've lost five pounds without much effort. Posture is one of the keys to becoming a fit female, and everything is connected. "The ankle bone's connected to the knee bone, the knee bone's connected to the hip bone. . . . " So, starting from the bottom and working your way up . . . if you wear high heels (which make you look fabulous, so why wouldn't you?), then you probably have tight ankles and other tight muscles up the chain, especially your lower back, which then leads to your upper body hunching forward to compensate. This, along with spending hours sitting at a desk, in the car, on the phone, or at the computer, leads to tight hip flexors and a more forward, rounded posture, which produces more of a slumped, frumpy look instead of a confident, sexy look. Incorporating stretches for your ankles, hip flexors, chest, and shoulders and foam rolling your upper and lower back to undo some of the postural dysfunctions your lifestyle creates will give you confident, tall posture to go with your new body and new attitude.

WHAT ABOUT YOGA?

If you enjoy yoga, it's a great way to get your stretch on. I have no problem with a fit female adding a yoga class to her schedule, *but* it does not replace a workout. I've found that yoga works great for stretching, quieting your mind, and providing cortisol reduction time, but over the long term, it will not turn you into a fit female. (Look around your yoga class.) The other downside is that a yoga class will stretch everything, so if you have a muscle group that's tighter than the others, take some extra time to stretch that area. For example, if your hip flexors are really tight and you go to yoga, you may stretch your hip flexors during class, but you'll also stretch everything else, so in relation, they'll still be your tightest muscles and will still have more tension in them than your other muscles do.

ONE OR TWO DAYS A WEEK, FOAM ROLL AND STRETCH FOR RECOVERY

In the beginning, you should go through the foam-rolling rituals at least two days a week. This will take you about 10 to 15 minutes. You can do it while you're watching TV. Instead of spending time on your couch, spend it on your foam roller. You may find that it's easiest to make it a habit every night before you go to bed. I put it on my clients' schedules one or two days a week at a minimum. I call it a foam-rolling ritual because it should become a ritual. Again, this is not optional.

FOAM ROLL DURING YOUR WORKOUTS

Foam rolling is listed at the end of each workout, too. This is the minimum you should do during a workout. If you find that you have a body part that's especially tight or sore, you may want to hop on the roller after you warm up but before you start your workout, to loosen everything up. You can also have a roller close by to use between sets, during your rest periods.

Below I list some of the different techniques you can try to get the most out of using your foam roller. Start doing the following and you'll know when you need to spend more time on one area than another.

FOAM-ROLLING RITUALS

Thoracic Mobilization

POSITION: Lying on the floor with the foam beneath your upper back and parallel to your shoulders, place your hands behind your head to support your neck. With your elbows out, roll your body slowly up and down over the roller as you extend and relax back onto it. You may get a chiropractic adjustment on this one, which should feel good.

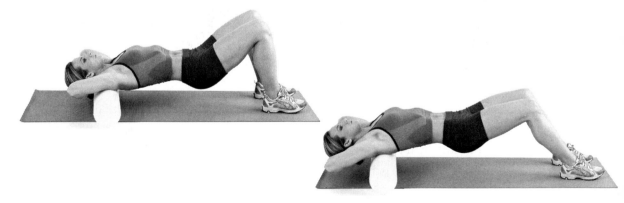

Hips

POSITION: Seated on the foam roller, cross your right leg over your left and lean toward your right hip, putting your weight on your right hand. Roll on your right gluteal muscle and stop if you feel a spot that feels like a knot. Switch sides and repeat.

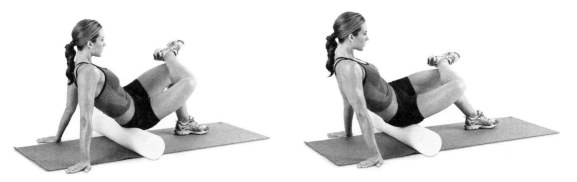

Hamstrings

POSITION: With your legs straight out with one leg crossed over the other to increase pressure. With your hands behind you and your weight resting on your arms, roll from the top of your right leg, at the point where your hamstring goes into your hip, all the way down to your knee. Put your weight on one leg and roll up and down, then switch legs and repeat.

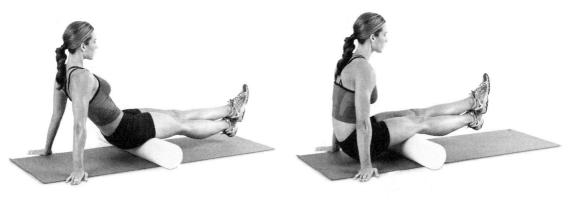

Calves

POSITION: This one will become your fave if you wear high heels a lot. From the same position as for your hamstrings, roll down so the roller is under your calves and, if you're up for it, cross one leg over the other and roll one calf at a time over the roller. If you can't handle that much weight, then do both calves at the same time.

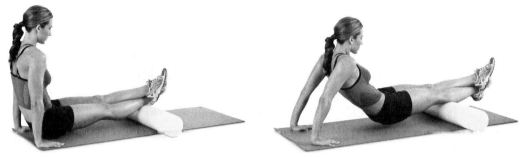

Iliotibial (IT) Band

POSITION: Turn on your right side so the roller is under the outer side of your right leg. Cross your left leg over so your left foot is flat on the floor and use it to push yourself up and down along the roller. Roll from your hip to your knee along the side of your right leg. Then repeat on your left leg. This one tends to hit a pretty sore spot, but you'll be glad you did it.

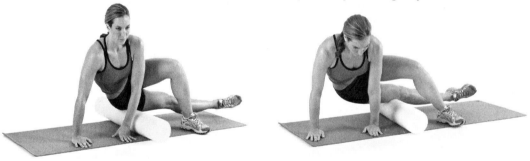

Quadriceps

POSITION: Turn face down so that the roller is underneath the tops of your thighs and lean to one side. Roll up and down, then lean to the other side and repeat.

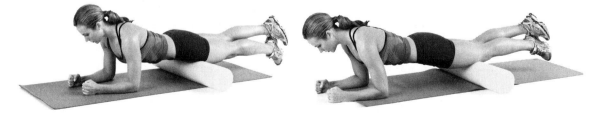

Latissimus Dorsi (Lats)

POSITION: Lie on the roller so that it's under your armpit and roll from your armpit to your hip, along the lat muscle. Then switch sides and repeat.

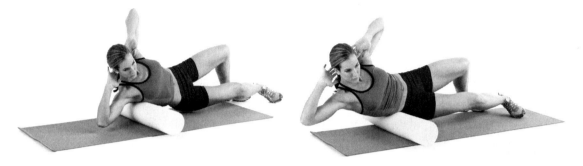

As you use your foam roller, you'll fall in love with it. It is the easiest, cheapest way to get a massage, and it will keep your muscles all feeling great. Use it regularly to avoid injury and feel great for your workouts!

STRETCHING RITUALS

Along with using a foam roller, you also need to make stretching a regular part of your routine. I've included many dynamic stretches in your warmup, but you should also spend some time doing static stretching. The phrase "If you don't use it, you lose it" rings true with regard to flexibility. After you spend 10 minutes on a foam roller, take five to 10 minutes to stretch.

Essential Stretching Guidelines

✦ **Sweat before you stretch:** For the best results, you should perform a good, solid warmup before doing any form of stretch-

ing. You *can* stretch cold, of course, but your results will be greatly enhanced if you break a sweat before you stretch.

✦ **Vary the stretching:** In addition to changing the order of the stretches and the types of stretches you do, you should also change the angle of pull with each stretch. For example, you can statically stretch your hamstring in several ways: One position that stretches the hamstring is lying on your back with, say, your right leg straight and raised from the hip, with or without the calf being stretched also (this will increase the hamstring stretch). You can do this with your leg pointed straight up, or you can take it across the midline of your body, toward the opposite side (in this case, the left). You can even move the leg out to the right, outside of your body. You can also turn your foot in or out as you perform the stretch. So you have two calf positions times three leg positions times two foot positions. That gives you *12* permutations of a lying-on-your-back hamstring stretch alone. The possibilities are literally endless and should be explored thoroughly. Every single adjustment will target different fibers.

♦ **Always stretch the tightest muscle or tightest side first:** As a general rule, a tight muscle will inhibit the stretch of all other muscles in the surrounding areas. It's a good idea to work on the worst areas first in the workout.

♦ **Stretch from the hips outward:** The sequence of stretching can dramatically improve your results. Stretching your hip flexors will reduce the anterior (forward) pull on your hips. This, in turn, will improve the range of motion of your hamstrings by reducing the tension on them. So you'll have increased range in a muscle group you have yet to stretch. This idea saves time and improves results—so always begin with the hip area and work outward.

♦ **Length of time:** An expert once told me that you should never hold a stretch for more than 15 seconds. Another expert told me you're wasting your time if you don't hold the stretch for at least 90 seconds. Someone else told me you just shouldn't stretch! What confusion! In my opinion, stretching is perhaps the only training activity of which more is better. I have *never* met anyone who I felt was spending too much time stretching (kind of like I've never met anyone who eats too many vegetables). Stretch more and eat more vegetables! I hold static stretches with my clients for two to three minutes. I increase the stretch or change the position slightly every 30 seconds or so.

Include the following stretches, but don't limit yourself to these:

Hip Flexor Stretch

The hip flexors are usually one of the tightest muscle groups, since, by nature, everything we do in life shortens the hip flexors—walking, sitting, climbing stairs, running.

Because they're attached to the back of the pelvis, having tight hip flexors will cause two things to happen:

1. Your hips will tilt forward, making it appear as if you have a bulging belly. This is very common on women who are in the Spinning cult. You know, the women who go to Spinning class every single morning at 5:00 A.M.? Spinning really tightens up your flexors, and if you look at any of these women as they walk out of a Spinning class, you'll notice they all have the top of

their hips tilted forward, with their butt sticking out, creating a pooch stomach that can easily be fixed by stopping the Spinning madness, stretching the hip flexors, and using a routine like the one in this book to get their butt switched on and working again.

2. The other problem that arises with tight hip flexors is lower-back pain. Because the hip flexors are attached at the back of the pelvis, when they're short, they pull the pelvis into anterior tilt, and this causes pressure at the lower back, where your body tries to compensate for the tight hip flexors.

Position: Stand on your left leg with your right foot resting on a step or chair behind you. Bend your left knee to lower yourself into a lunge until your right knee is resting on the floor. Lunge forward, pushing your hips forward and keeping your torso upright. You should feel a stretch in the front of your right hip. To intensify the stretch, turn your body away from your right leg or raise your right arm straight up over your head and lean away from your right leg. Switch legs and repeat.

Glute/Hip Stretch

There are a couple of different ways to stretch your hips, all of which include having the leg you're stretching at a 90-degree angle from your torso. You can face a table and lay your leg on the table at a 90-degree angle from your body, or even sit and cross your leg over, the

way a man crosses his legs, and use your hands to put light pressure on your knee. The move shown here is called the 90/90 stretch, because each leg should be at a 90-degree angle.

Position: Sit on the floor with your right leg at a 90-degree angle in front of you and your left leg at a 90-degree angle behind you. Keep your back flat as you walk your hands forward and feel a stretch in your hip. Repeat on the other side.

Posterior Chain/ Hamstring Stretch

This stretches your entire posterior chain, including your back, hamstrings, and calves.

Position: Lying on your back, start with a hamstring stretch with a towel or jump rope looped around your foot and pulling your leg toward you, keeping the knee straight. After your hamstring has stretched some, take the leg across your body, keeping your torso face up, and pull your leg up along your body as high as you can, keeping your other leg still. Repeat on the other side.

Chest Stretch

This is an excellent stretch for most women, who tend to have forward, rounded posture. This stretch opens up your chest and undoes what you probably do all day, which is round forward. Doing this stretch can help alleviate neck tension that has built up from being on the computer or the phone.

Position: Stand close to a wall or in a

doorway and, with your arm extended horizontally at a 90-degree angle from your shoulder and braced against the wall or door frame, turn your torso away until you feel a stretch in your chest. Or lie on the floor with your foam roller under your spine, supporting your head. Relax your arms out to the sides, feeling a stretch in your chest. Slowly bend your elbows up to a 90-degree angle to isolate the stretch even more.

Don't forget, as we discussed in Fit Female Credo Secret #7, you need to make R, R & R a priority! As you are becoming a fit female, be sure to make these recovery and regeneration rituals a part of your routine: Get your sleep, always have a postworkout shake, foam roll regularly, and stretch your muscles. Be good to your body and it will be good back to you.

FIT FEMALE *Real Life Story*

▲
Janelle before

▶
Janelle lost 18 pounds of fat and 2 clothing sizes.

I *look* better. That's a great accomplishment—getting my self-confidence back. I'm very happy with how I look now.

✦ I learned that dieting really isn't that difficult. It's mostly about portion control.

✦ I am not afraid of cookies.

✦ I like exercising. I feel great afterward.

I'm so happy to be getting my old body back. Except I'm *strong* now, besides being thinner. I admire strong bodies, not those waiflike model bodies. Try being pregnant on a frame like that—not possible. ✦

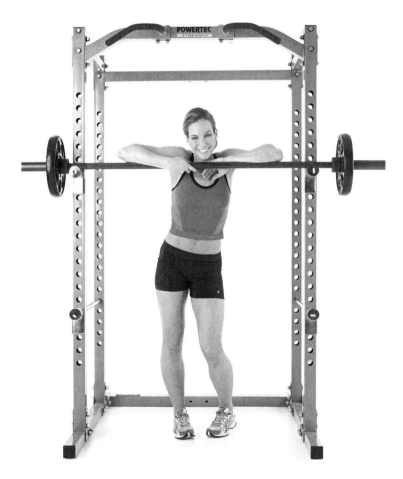

WRAPPING IT UP

Chapter 13

Maintaining Your New Body

Are your friends calling you a BITCH yet? Have you become inspiring, totally confident, and hot? Are you turning heads at the grocery store? Do you feel sexy wearing anything you throw on? Are you empowered? Fit? Fabulous?

You did it! You are a fit female! Time to embrace and enjoy your new fit chick body and lifestyle and start to feed off inspiring others! That's right, guaranteed, you will have people come up to you and say, "You look great!" "What do you do?" "Are you an athlete?" They want to know the secrets you know to become fit and fabulous. They see your confidence and how good you feel in your own skin, and *that* is what they want to find for themselves. When you start to inspire others, you have come full circle. Congratulations—from one fit female to another!

Having a goal gives you a direction to go in and helps you to know whether you are on the right path. Setting and reaching a goal is one thing, but maintaining the goal is everything. Few people who successfully lose weight or change their bodies can maintain their new physiques. In fact, 95 percent of people who lose weight gain it back again within 12 months. Typically, weight loss causes decreases in lean body mass and resting metabolism, which makes it very easy to regain the lost weight.

However, your fit journey has been completely different from the journey the average person takes to achieve the body they want. And that, my fit friend, is why you also will not gain the fat back, the way the average person does. You have completely reinvented yourself! In fact, as I mentioned at the start of your journey, the number on the scale may not

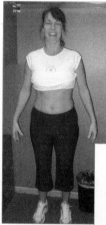

▲
Nina, before, came in covering up in her T-shirt and long pants.

Nina lost 10 pounds of fat and ▶ transformed her body.

FIT FEMALE *Real life Story*

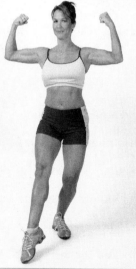

I have been exercising in one way or another for most of my life. It started at age 3 with downhill skiing, gymnastics, and ballet till age 14. Then there was the late-'70s craze of high-impact aerobics (oh, how that hurt my knees!), plus running, NordicTrack, treadmills, Total Gyms, Nautilus machines, Curves Gym, and other fitness clubs—specifically the kind that offer little to *no* assistance. As far back as I can remember, I have been very weight conscious and truly *never* satisfied with my body. This has been a constant struggle and a painful experience. Emotionally, it tore at me until I felt hopeless and struggled with bouts of binge eating and throwing up during my college years. Fortunately, I was able to get away from this behavior of bingeing and purging—really not sure how, but I did!

However, in my head I still felt trapped in an ugly, dumpy-looking body. Funny thing is, I never really was more than five to 10 pounds overweight. Now, looking back, I know I was not overweight. Instead, I had no muscle tone whatsoever! I really was a flabby mess! Clothes could hide all that, so I kept doing whatever ineffective exercising I was doing and lived feeling completely dissatisfied with my body.

have changed very much, but who cares? You're wearing your thermometer jeans and are looking *hot*! You have boosted your metabolism to the point where it is sizzling and you can't miss a meal because you'll be too hungry. Your body burns through everything so fast now, you can't imagine running on empty! You have increased your lean body mass, which further stokes your metabolism. By now, lifting weights is part of your lifestyle, and pushing yourself in the gym to get even stronger and more fit is a way of life.

Weight training helps preserve muscle mass and resting metabolism and will make it easy to keep your fit and fabulous new figure. Don't believe me? Research from the University of Alabama at Birmingham studied the effects of losing 26 pounds on lean body mass, body fat, and resting metabolic rate in women participating in a weight-loss program. Women either

---

Back in 2004, I was eating breakfast at a local restaurant and happened to notice a man and woman come in to eat in workout clothes. They must have worked together, because their shirts had the same logo. I specifically remember how buff the woman was. I was so impressed with both of their physiques that it was hard to stop staring! They ate breakfast and left the restaurant. I noticed that they walked into a local gym across the street; it was then that I knew I had to check it out. I was surprised to find out there were no machines, just free weights and personal trainers who worked with you on a training program. I was getting remarried in six months, and I really wanted to look my best. I joined the gym for a three-month trial membership, and I'm still there today—four years later! It was by far the *best* thing I have ever done for myself.

I have never felt so good about myself. I've changed the way I look by building muscle and losing body fat. I never would have thought that heavy weight training would help me achieve not only a better body but a much more positive self-image. That pain I experienced for years is gone. At age 48, I now look at myself and feel good about me. I still have my moments when I feel dissatisfied about the way I look, but I must say they are short-lived! It actually motivates me to work out harder and eat cleaner. That sure beats bingeing and purging. I feel more confident and have started to accept compliments without putting myself down. There's nothing worse than someone saying something nice to you and all you do is deny it. No more!

I now train five days a week—three days of resistance training and two days of kettlebell classes—and feel like it is therapy for me. Now that I'm in my forties, I know that if I stop training, I'll lose muscle mass and gain fat. I realize how important weight training is to maintain a healthy body. I'll never stop! I am so grateful for that day when I watched the two trainers go into that small gym. It has changed my life for good! ✦

lifted weights, did aerobics, or did no exercise. The women who weight-trained during the weight-loss program were able to sustain lean body mass and maintain resting metabolic rate compared with the women who didn't exercise or did aerobics. Combining caloric restriction with weight training results in long-lasting weight loss.

The truth is, life can be stressful and complicated, and things will come up to keep you from being your optimal fit female self all the time. It's important to set realistic goals and find a middle ground between the ultimate physical appearance and what is realistic for your lifestyle, and at the same time easy to maintain. The body you are happiest in, feel good in, and can wear whatever you want in but can still live life to the fullest and not feel deprived or restricted. Concentrate on achieving a healthier appearance, feeling good about yourself, and being fit, confident, and fabulous.

Reread the Fit Female Credo and live by it every day!

The key is not to throw out everything you've learned and go back to your old ways. Stick with what has worked to get you to your new body. Eat exactly as you've been eating on this program. Don't all of a sudden, because you are at your goal, change everything that has been working up until this point. Give yourself room to enjoy yourself, but stay within the guidelines most of the time and continue making healthy choices. Keep giving your body what it's become accustomed to during your fit female journey.

You will not be perfect all the time. Expecting perfection will only set you up for failure. Studies have shown that people who are flexible dieters (as opposed to rigid dieters) tend to weigh less, maintain better adherence to their diets in the long run, and have fewer binge-eating episodes. Now that you are where you want to be, you can get away with sticking to the rules 90 percent of the time and allowing yourself to relax 20 percent of the time. You probably won't take this whole 20 percent most weeks if your body has become used to the fit female program, but when the holidays arrive, you know you can enjoy yourself. You know how to stay in control and stick to your plan 90 percent of the time, but look out on Thanksgiving, because you'll be helping yourself to some brown-sugar-covered sweet potatoes and some pumpkin pie. And you'll enjoy it and get back to your usual eating habits the next day. Because you can! The 80 percent rule means you can allow yourself one meal or even one whole day completely off your usual healthy plan once a week to eat whatever you want. This will give you room for special occasions and unexpected outings. You don't have to live in a bubble to maintain your new physique. Don't beat yourself up because you had a piece of cake at a birthday party or ate some bread when you went out to dinner. Instead savor it, but get right back on track later in the day, or the next day.

Your body will fluctuate. There will be times of the year when you'll eat a little more and your body fat will be a little higher. Enjoy yourself and center your holidays around the people you're with, rather than food. Don't deprive yourself of your mother's homemade pie or your grandma's sweet potatoes if those are things you've always looked forward to on those special occasions. Instead, help yourself to a small portion and take pleasure in the people around you. Enjoy life and enjoy feeling fit and fabulous!

Keep your thermometer jeans close by at all times. If you start taking one too many cheat meals or even just having an extra 100 calories here and there, it will add up—and those jeans will let you know, believe me! Keep an eye on how your clothes feel and what your measurements say, and if you reach the point where you have to lie on your bed to put your jeans on because they've gotten too tight, it's time to take immediate action to get back to where you were. You know what clothing size and degree of body fat make you feel and look good. You also know how much hard work you put in to get there. A simple way to maintain your new body is to keep those jeans fitting well. Don't make any exceptions. You must immediately get back on track when you see yourself creeping close to your upper limit. Don't let another day go by without taking action.

Let's review how you'll maintain your new fit female body:

1. Don't throw out everything you've learned and go back to your old ways. Stick with what worked to get you to your new body. Eat exactly as you have been eating. Sure, you've changed your body, and that's great, but what you've also changed is your lifestyle. This is how you live now.

2. Be flexible. Give yourself room to splurge, but get right back on track. Don't beat yourself up. Allow yourself one splurge meal or one day off from the nutrition rules each week. The rest of the week, stick to what got you here in the first place. Remember the 90 percent rule for maintenance.

3. Watch out for your trigger foods. You know which foods send you into a frenzy of gorging on junk. Stay away from them. If you have certain foods that trigger you, avoid eating them.

4. Give yourself a range within which to stay, and don't make any exceptions. The day your jeans start to feel snug is the day you need to get back on track to your goal. Throw away all your "fat" jeans and clothes; you don't want them there to tempt you. Do not keep your fat clothes! Give them away!

To keep yourself motivated with new workouts and advice (along with direct access to me), join the Fit Female Community at thefemalebodybreakthrough.com where you can trade notes and stories with other fit females just like you!

Chapter 14

The Fit Female Journey Continues...

What a journey you have been on! By now, if you've followed this plan, you've become inspiring, totally confident, and hot—you are the BITCH. And now that you understand the new meaning of the word, you can be proud of being one. Enjoy the benefits of your new way of life—unstoppable energy, confidence, strength, optimal health, improved self-esteem, fulfilling relationships, and, above all, that fit and sexy feeling.

The gym is now your domain as much as any man's. You should be using food as fuel to keep your metabolism revving high. One woman at a time, we are taking over the training floor, fueling our bodies for great workouts instead of starving ourselves to get the bodies we want.

You've worked hard to get where you are, so keep up your workout schedule day after day, week after week, month after month. Don't be afraid to push yourself harder in the gym. Lift weights that challenge you consistently and exercise with an attitude of what you *can* do, not what you can't. Don't get what we call around our gym, the "C word" or complacent. Keep moving forward by setting new goals, taking on new challenges, and pushing yourself to maintain your fit female body.

Beware: You will be a role model for others and you might inspire a future fit female. Women will be coming to you for advice and motivation. By all means, share your secrets—and this book! Start a dialogue about what to eat, how to work out, and how to keep an inspired, motivated mindset. Before long you'll be encouraging each other to stay on the plan and continue challenging your bodies.

To continue your journey, you and your fellow fit females can get ongoing support from me, your coach, at thefemalebodybreakthrough.com. You can join the community of fit females to share your story, get inspiration from other fit females, and trade tips for meals, motivational strategies, and workouts. Ladies, your journey to a fit and healthy life style has only just begun!

Acknowledgments

To all of my clients, the original fit females, who have trusted me with their bodies over the years: Thank you for believing in me and letting me be a part of each of your life transformations. I have learned so much from each and every one of you. I was able to gain hands-on experience to write this book thanks to you.

Also, a huge thank you to all of the fitness professionals and colleagues, many of whom I also consider good friends. I have been very fortunate to learn from them and continue to learn from them in this industry, and many (but not all) are named throughout the book. With their influence, they have helped me to form my own philosophies.

Thank you to the personal development gurus including: Jim Rohn, Brian Tracey, Zig Ziglar, Anthony Robbins, and Bob Proctor, who have all had a huge influence in helping me to create my own positive mindset, and to go after and accomplish what I want in life. Through their books and courses, I have learned their philosophies and transformed my own mindset and the mindset of many of my clients.

Thank you to Thomas Plummer who gave me the advice to "Learn more about one thing and be the best at it. Your one thing should be how to train women."

Also thank you to Adam Campbell who answered my endless e-mails and phone calls giving me the encouragement, reassurance, and advice I needed as a first-time rookie author, helping me to make sure my photo shoot went smoothly, and teaching me all of the veteran photo shoot tricks.

Thank you to the Results Fitness team. Without your help and support I never could have written this book. Thank you for your patience throughout this book-writing process. I especially want to thank Mike Wunsch, Craig Rasmussen, Joe Hand, and Cameron Hedges, who all played a part in coaching the women in this book. And a huge thank you to Donna Bent, who keeps our gym running like a well-oiled machine and was one of the fit females who gave me inspiration for this book. I could not have done this without you. You are the best there is! I count on you guys every single day to make our gym the best it can be, and I appreciate every one of you and what you contribute.

Thank you, Courtney Conroy. Your trust and belief in me gave me the confidence and inspiration to write this book. I appreciate your letting me have the freedom to be creative, and giving me the guidance I needed to make this book the best it can be.

To my family who have always believed in me: Special thanks to my mom and dad, who have always encouraged me to follow my dreams, have focused on my strengths, and have given me unconditional support. You helped me form my beliefs about who I am and what I am capable of. I owe my passion for fitness to my dad, who got me hooked on the gym and working out when I was young. Thanks, Dad! And to my mom for always being there for me and being my best friend throughout my life.

To my grandma, who is my biggest fan and always has been: Thank you for your ongoing encouragement and, of course, all of your bragging.

Thank you to Alwyn—my husband, my superhero, my best friend, and my soul mate—for always raising the bar for me and believing in me more than I believe in myself. Together we accomplish so much more than I could ever dream of accomplishing on my own. You truly bring out the best in me. I appreciate your patience throughout this book-writing process, reading the book over and over . . . and over again, and even being a good sport trying out the fit female program and credo yourself. This book is our book, with our ideas, philosophies, and programs that we have shaped together. Thank you for letting me bounce ideas off you, giving me feedback, and encouraging me to create a book that is "really what we do" at our gym. I would not be where I am without you.

And, above all, I thank the Lord in whom I put my faith, and who has surrounded me with such amazing, supportive people in my life. I am truly blessed.

References

Chapter 1

Strength training better than aerobics

Hunter, G.R., Byrne, N.M., Sirikul, B., Fernández, J.R., Zuckerman, P.A., Darnell, B.E., and Gower, B.A. 2008. Resistance training conserves fat-free mass and resting energy expenditure following weight loss. *Obesity* (Silver Spring) 16(5):1045–51. Epub 2008 Mar 6.

Stress

Chek, Paul. 2004. CHEK Institute, Nutrition and Lifestyle Coaching Certification.

Epel, E.S., McEwen, B., Seeman, T., Matthews, K., Castellazzo, G., Brownell, K.D., Bell, J., and Ickovics, J.R. 2000. Stress and body shape: stress-induced cortisol secretion is consistently greater among women with central fat. *Psychosomatic Medicine* 62:623–632.

Sapolsky, Robert. 1998. *Why Zebras Don't Get Ulcers.* W.H. Freeman.

Sleep

Redwine, L., Hauger, R.L., Gillin, J.C., and Irwin, M. 2000. Effects of sleep and sleep deprivation on interleukin-6, growth hormone, cortisol, and melatonin levels in humans. *J Clin Endocrinol Metab* 85(10):3597–603.

Wiley, T.S. 2000. *Lights Out.* Simon & Schuster.

Smoking

Archives of Dermatological Research. April 2000 292:188.

Brix, T.H., Hansen, P.S., Kyvik, K.O., and Hegedüs, L. 2000. Cigarette smoking and risk of clinically overt thyroid disease: a population-based twin case-control study. *Arch Intern Med* 160(5):661–66.

Department of Health and Human Services Center for Disease Control and Prevention. Women and Smoking. Surgeon General's Report, 2001.

Television watching

Neilsen Company. Quarterly Media Report. 770 Broadway New York, NY 10003-9595.

50,000 thoughts a day

National Science Foundation. 4201 Wilson Boulevard, Arlington, Virginia 22230; http://www.nsf.gov/index.jsp.

Rohn, Jim. 2002. *One Year Success Plan Course.* Jim Rohn International.

Chapter 2

National Weight Control Registry Brown Medical School/The Miriam Hospital Weight Control & Diabetes Research Center, 196 Richmond Street, Providence, RI 02903.

Chapter 3

Braun, W.A., Hawthorne, W.E., and Markofski, M.M. 2005. Acute EPOC response in women to circuit training and treadmill exercise of matched oxygen consumption. *Eur Journ Applied Physiology* 94(5-6):500–504.

Bryner, R.W., Ullrich, I.H., Sauers, J., Donley, D., Hornsby, G., Kolar, M., and Yeater, R. 1999. Effects of resistance vs. aerobic training combined with an 800 calorie liquid diet on lean body mass and resting metabolic rate. *J Am Coll Nutr.* 18(2):115–21.

Nindl, B.C., Harman, E.A., Marx, J.O., Gotshalk, L.A., Frykman, P.N., Lammi, E., Palmer, C., and Kraemer, W.J. 2000. Regional body composition changes in women after 6 months of periodized physical training. *Journal of Applied Physiology* 88(6):2251–59.

Rana, S.R., Chleboun, G.S., Gilders, R.M., Hagerman, F.C., Herman, J.R., Hikida, R.S., Kushnick, M.R., Staron, R.S., and Toma, K. 2008. Comparison of early phase adaptations for traditional strength and endurance, and low velocity resistance training programs in college-aged women. *J Strength Cond Res* 22(1):119–27.

Velthuis, M.J., Schuit, A.J., Peeters, P.H., and Monninkhof, E.M. 2009. Exercise program affects body composition but not weight in postmenopausal women. *Menopause* Feb 2.

Bone mass increases

Cussler, Lohman et al. 2003. Weight lifted in strength training predicts bone change in postmenopausal women. *Med Sci Sports Exerc.* 35(1):10–7.

Nickols-Richardson, S.M., Miller, L.E., Wooten, D.F., Ramp W.K., and Herbert, W.G. 2007. Concentric and Eccentric isokinetic resistance training similarly increases muscular strength, fat free tissue mass and specific bone mineral measurements in young women. *Osteoporosis Int.* 18(6):789-96.

Winters, K.M. and Snow, C.M. 2000. Detraining reverses positive effects of exercise on the musculoskeletal system in premenopausal women. *J Bone Miner Res.* (12):2495-503.

Decrease risk of injuries

Myer, G.D., Ford, K.R., Brent, J.L., and Hewett, T.E. 2007. Differential neuromuscular training effects on ACL injury risk factors in "high risk" verses "low risk" athletes. *BMC Musculoskeletal Disord.* 8:39.

Boost stamina and function in everyday activities

Hartman, M.J., Fields, D.A., Byrne, N.M., and Hunter, G. R. 2007. Resistance training improves metabolic economy during functional tasks in older adults. *Journal of Strength and Conditioning Research* 21(1):91–95.

Aging

Koopman, R., and L.J. Van Loon. 2009. Aging, exercise and muscle protein metabolism. *Journal of Applied Physiology* 106(6):2040–8. Epub 2009 Jan 8.

Kravitz, Len, Ph.D. 2009. The Female Training Advantages (lecture, ECA Conference).

Melov, S., Tarnopolsky, M.A., Beckman, K., Felkey, K., and Hubbard, A. 2007. Resistance exercise reverses aging in human skeletal muscle. *PLoS ONE* 2(5):e465.

Dictionary, definition of metabolism

www.dictionary.com

Strength training won't make you big and bulky

Brown, et al. 1974. The effects of maximal resistance training on the strength and body composition of women athletes. *Med Sci Sports Exerc.* 6(3):174–77.

Kravitz, Len, Ph.D. 2009. The Female Training Advantages (lecture, ECA Conference).

Marx, J.O., et al. 2001. Low-volume circuit versus high-volume periodized resistance training in women. *Med Sci Sports Exerc.* 33(4):635–43.

Aerobics is all you need

Kraemer, W.J., et al. 2001. Resistance training combined with bench step aerobics enhances women's health profile. *Med Sci Sports Exerc.* 33(2):259–69.

Aerobics ineffective for fat loss

Kramer, W.J., et al. 1999. Influence of exercise training on physiological and performance changes with weight loss in men. *Med. Sci Sports Exerc.* 31(9):1320–1329.

McTiernan, A., et al. 2007. Exercise effect on weight and body fat in men and women. *Obesity* (Silver Spring) 15(6):1496–512.

Redman, L.M., et al. 2007. Effect of calorie restriction with or without exercise on body composition and fat distribution. *J Clin Endocrinol Metab.* 92(3):865-72. Epub 2007 Jan 2.

Schuenke, M.D., Mikat, R.P., and McBride, J.M. 2002. Effect of an acute period of resistance exercise on excess post-exercise oxygen consumption: implications for body mass management. *Eur J Appl Physiol.* 86(5):411–7. Epub 2002 Jan 29.

Stokes, K.A., Nevill, M.E., Hall, G.M., and Lakomy, H. K. 2002. The time course of the human growth hormone response to a 6 s and a 30 s cycle ergometer sprint. *J Sports Sci.* 20(6):487-94.

Talanian, Galloway, et al. 2006. Two weeks of high intensity aerobic interval training increases the capacity for fat oxidation during exercise in women. *J Appl Physiol.* 102(4):1439–47. Epub 2006 Dec 14.

Trapp, E.G., Chisholm, D.J., Freund, J., and Boutcher, S.H. 2008. The effects of high intensity intermittent exercise training on fat loss and fasting insulin levels of young women. *Int J Obesity* 32(4):684–91.

Tremblay, A., Simoneau, J.A., and Bouchard, C. 1994. Impact of exercise intensity on body fatness and skeletal muscle metabolism. *Metabolism* 43(7):814–8.

Utter, A.C., Nieman, D.C., et al. 1998 Influence of diet and/or exercise on body composition and cardio respiratory fitness in obese women. *Int J Sport Nutr.* 8(3):213–22.

Chapter 4

Maltz, Maxwell, M.D., F.I.C.S. 1960. *Psychocybernetics.* Simon & Schuster.

Rohn, Jim. 2002. *One Year Success Plan Course.* Jim Rohn International.

Tracey, Brian. 2004 *Goals!* Berrett-Koheler Publishers.

Chapter 5

Robbins, Anthony. 1991. *Awaken the Giant Within.* Simon & Schuster.

Chapter 6

Menstrual cycle

Seeley, Rod, Stephens, Trent, and Philip Tate. 1991. *Essentials of Anatomy and Physiology.* Mosby-Year Book 502–507.

Performance and mood affected by cycle

Eston, R.G., et al. 1984. The regular menstrual cycle and athletic performance. *Sports Med.* 1(6):431–45.

Middleton, L.E. and H.A. Wenger. 2006. Effects of menstrual phase on performance and recovery in intense intermittent activity. *Eur J Appl Physiol.* 96(1):53–58. Epub 2005 Oct 26.

Petrofsky, J., Al Malty, A., and Suh, H.J. 2007. Isometric endurance, body and skin temperature and limb and skin blood flow during menstrual cycle. *Med Sci Monit.* 13(3):CR111–117.

Williams, T.J. and G.S. Krahenbuhl. 1997. Menstrual cycle phase and running economy. *Med Sci Sports Exerc.* 29(12):1609–18.

Burning fat for fuel during menstruation

D'Eon, T. and B. Braun. 2002. The roles of estrogen and progesterone in regulating carbohydrate and fat utilization at rest and during exercise. *J Womens Health Gend Based Med.* 11(3):225-37.

D'Eon, T.M., Sharoff, C., Chipkin, S.R., Grow, D., Ruby, B.C., and Braun, B. 2002. Regulation of exercise carbohydrate metabolism by estrogen and progesterone in women. *Am J Physiol Endocrinol Metab.* 283(5): E1046–55.

Dye, L. and J.E. Blundell. 1997. Menstrual cycle and appetite control: implications for weight regulation. *Hum Reprod.* 12(6):1142–51.

Heiling, V.J. and M.D. Jensen.1992. Free fatty acid metabolism in the follicular and luteal phases of the menstrual cycle. *J Clin Endocrinol Metab.* 74(4):806–10.

Jacobs, Kevin A., Casazza, Gretchen A., Suh, Sang-Hoon, Horning, Michael A., and Brooks, George A. 2004. Fatty acid reesterification but not oxidation is increased by oral contraceptive use in women. *J Appl Physiol.* 98:1720–1731. Epub 2004 Dec 23.

Jahromi, M.K., Gaeini, A., and Rahimi, Z. 2008. Influence of a physical fitness course on menstrual cycle characteristics. *Gynecol Endocrinol.* 24(11):659–62.

Petrofsky, J., Al Malty, A., and Suh, H.J. 2007. Isometric endurance, body and skin temperature and limb and skin blood flow during the menstrual cycle. *Med Sci Monit.* 13(3):CR111–7.

Serrano, Eric, M.D. 1999. The War on Fat Seminar.

Chapter 8

Eat breakfast

Jakubowicz, M.D. of Hospital de Clinicias, et al. June 2008. Virginia Commonwealth University, Caracas, Venezuela.

Meal frequency

Farshchi, H.R., Taylor, M.A., and MacDonald, I.A. 2004. Decreased thermic effect of food after an irregular compared with a regular meal pattern in healthy lean women. *Int J Obes Related Metab Disord.* 28(5):653–60.

Iwao, S., Mori, K., and Sato, Y. 1996. Effects of meal frequency on body composition during weight control in boxers. *Scand J Med Sci Sports* 6(5):265–72.

Louis-Sylvestre, J., Lluch, A., Neant, F., and Blundell, J. E. 2003. Highlighting the positive impact of increasing feeding frequency on metabolism and weight management. *Forum Nutr.* 56:126–28. Review.

Eat protein

Frestedt, J.L., Zenk, J.L., Kuskowski, M.A., Ward, L.S., and Bastian, E.D. 2008. A whey protein supplement increases fat loss and spares lean muscle in obese subjects: a randomized human clinical study. *Nutr Metab (Lond).* 5:8.

Krieger, J.W., Sitren, H.S., Daniels, M.J., and Langkamp-Henken, B. 2006. Effects of variation in protein and carbohydrate intake on body mass and composition during energy restriction. *Am J Clin Nutr.* 83(2):260–74.

Vander Wal, J.S., Gupta, A., Khosla, P., Dhurandhar, N. V. 2008. Egg breakfast enhances weight loss. *Int J Obes (Lond).* 32(10):1545–51. Epub 2008 Aug 5.

Eliminate processed carbohydrates

Yancy, William S., Jr., Olsen, Maren K., Guyton, John R., Bakst, Ronna P., and Westman, Eric C. 2004. A low-carbohydrate, ketogenic diet versus a low-fat diet to treat obesity and hyperlipidemia. *Annals of Internal Medicine* 140(10):769–77.

Water

Stookey, J.D., Constant, F., Popkin, B.M., and Gardner, C.D. 2008. Drinking water is associated with weight loss in overweight dieting women independent of diet and activity. *Obesity (Silver Spring).* 16(11):2481–8. Epub 2008 Sep 11.

Caffeine

Acheson, K.J., Zahorska-Markiewicz, B., Pittet, P.H., Anantharaman, K., and Jéquier, E. 1980. Caffeine and coffee: their influence on metabolic rate and substrate utilization in normal and obese individuals. *Am J Clin Nutr.* 33:989–97.

Dulloo, A.G., Geisler, C.A., Horton, T., Collins, A., and Miller, D.S. 1989. Normal caffeine consumption: influence on thermogenesis and daily energy expenditure in lean and postobese human volunteers. *Am J Clin Nutr.* 49:44–50.

Shixian, Q., VanCrey, B., Shi, J., Kakuda, Y., and Jiang, Y. 2006. Green tea extract thermogenesis-induced weight loss by epigallocatechin gallate inhibition of catechol-O-methyltransferase. *Journal Medicinal Foods* 9:451–458.

Venables, M.C., Hulston, C.J., Cox, H.R., and Jeukendrup, A.E. 2008. Green tea extract ingestion, fat oxidation, and glucose tolerance in healthy humans. *American Journal Nutrition* 87:778–784.

Fish oil supplements

Hill, A.M., Buckley, J.D., Murphy, K.J., and Howe, P.R. 2007. Combining fish-oil supplements with regular aerobic exercise improves body composition and cardiovascular disease risk factors. *American Journal of Clinical Nutrition* 85:1267–1274.

Hill, A.M., Worthley, C., Murphy, K.J., Buckley, J.D., Ferrante, A., and Howe, P.R. 2007. n-3 fatty acid supplementation and regular moderate exercise: differential effects of a combined intervention on neutrophil function. *British Journal of Nutrition* 98:300–309.

Post workout shake

Berardi, J.M., Price, T.B., Noreen, E.E., and Lemon, P.W. 2006. Post exericse muscle glycogen recovery enhanced with carbohydrate-protein supplement. *Med Sci Sports Exerc.* 38(6):1106–13.

Chapter 9

Increase fish intake

Couet, C., Delarue, J., Ritz, P., Antoine, J.M., and Lamisse, F. 1997. Effect of dietary fish oil on body fat mass and basal fat oxidation in healthy adults. *Int J Obes Relat Metab Disord.* 21(8):637–43.

Chapter 10

Core first in program

Leetun, T.T., et al. 2004. Core stability measures as risk factors for lower extremity injury in athletes. *Med. Sci. Sports Exerc.* 36(6):926–934.

Simão, R., Farinatti Pde, T., Polito, M.D., Viveiros, L., and Fleck, S.J. 2007. Influence of exercise order on the number of repetitions performed and perceived exertion during resistance exercise in women. *Journal of Strength and Conditioning Research* 21(1): 23–28.

Pelvic floor disorder

Bø, K. 2006. Can pelvic floor muscle training prevent and treat pelvic organ prolapse? *Acta Obstet Gynecol Scand.* 85(3):263–8.

Dietz, H.P. 2008. Prolapse worsens with age, doesn't it? *Aust N Z J Obstet Gynaecol* 48(6):587–91.

Hay-Smith, E.J., Bø, K., Berghmans, L.C., Hendriks, H.J., de Bie, R.A., and van Waalwijk van Doorn, E.S. 2007. Pelvic floor muscle training for urinary incontinence in women. *Cochrane Database Syst Rev.* (1): CD001407.

Nygaard, I., Barber, M.D., Burgio, K.L., Kenton, K., Meikle, S., Schaffer, J., Spino, C., Whitehead, W.E., Wu, J., and Brody, D.J. 2008. Prevalence of symptomatic pelvic floor disorders in US women. *Pelvic Floor Disorders Network* 300(11):1311–16.

Women use fat for fuel during exercise but burn fat more slowly

Tarnopolsky, M.A. 2000. Gender differences in substrate metabolism during endurance exercise. *Can J Appl Physiology* 25(4):312–27.

Chapter 12

Post workout nutrition–3-4:1 ratio

Kerksick, C., et al. 2008. International Society of Sports Nutrition position stand: nutrient timing. *Journal of the International Society of Sports Nutrition* 5:17.

Chapter 13

Strength training to increase metabolism

Hunter, G.R., Byrne, N.M., Sirikul, B., Fernández, J.R., Zuckerman, P.A., Darnell, B.E., and Gower, B.A. 2008. Resistance training conserves fat-free mass and resting energy expenditure following weight loss. *Obesity* (Silver Spring) 16(5):1045–51. Epub 2008 Mar 6.

95-98% of people gain weight back

Leibel, Rudolph, M.D. 2004. Obesity: A diesase, not a character flaw. Lecture presented in the Grand Rounds Great Teachers Lecture series at the National Institutes of Health, Bethesda, MD.

Rigid dieters vs. flexible dieters

Stewart, T.M., Williamson, D.A., and White, M.A. 2002. Rigid vs. flexible dieting: association with eating disorder symptoms in nonobese women. *Appetite* 38(1):39–44.

Smith, C.F., Williamson, D.A., Bray, G.A., and Ryan, D.H. 1999. Flexible vs. rigid dieting strategies: relationship with adverse behavioral outcomes. *Appetite* 32(3):295–305.

Index

Underscored page references indicate sidebars and tables. **Boldface** references indicate photographs.